UNIVE'

DRIl

This book m
self servic
Fin

Stroboscopy

and Other Techniques for the Analysis of Vocal Fold Vibration

Stroboscopy

and Other Techniques for the Analysis of Vocal Fold Vibration

Gerhard Boehme MD, PhD
Technical University of Munich

and

Manfred Gross MD, PhD
Free University and the Humboldt University of Berlin

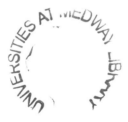

W

WHURR PUBLISHERS
LONDON AND PHILADELPHIA

© 2005 Whurr Publishers

First Published 2005
Whurr Publishers Ltd
19b Compton Terrace, London N1 2UN, England and
325 Chestnut Street, Philadelphia PA19106, USA

British Library Cataloguing in Publication Data
A catalogue record for this book is available from the
British Library.

ISBN 1 86156 384 1

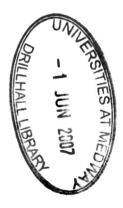

Printed and bound in the UK by
Henry Ling Limited, at the Dorset Press

Contents

Introduction

Laryngostroboscopy is the process by which the normal and pathological vibrating processes of the vocal folds are made visible during phonation.

The technique is a testing method used worldwide within both laryngology and phoniatric practice.

It is a technique normally undertaken by Ear, Nose and Throat specialists, but in some countries it is also used by speech-language pathologists/therapists.

Intensive training is required to use laryngostroboscopy effectively when carrying out differential diagnostic tests using stroboscopy. This book describes the theoretical background and clinical uses of the method for the evaluation of organic, functional and psychogenic laryngeal disorders.

This book serves both as an introduction to the subject for those new to the technique and a manual for those refining their skills.

Acknowledgements

We should like to thank our colleagues Professor F. Sram, MD and J.G. Svec, PhD (Prague) warmly for the generous provision of interesting image material and discussions on the value of video kymography. Also deserving of thanks is Professor W. Behrendt, MD (Leipzig) who provided us with histological findings on organic voice disorders. We were also able to integrate findings successfully from the histological collection of Professor O. Kleinsasser, MD (Marburg), compiled by Senior Physician N. Kleinsasser, MD (Munich), into our text. We thank Professor U. Eysholdt, MD for the critical overview of the section on high-speed cinematography.

We thank Mrs E. Kater for her tireless efforts in drafting the text in electronic form. Mr B. Dautert kindly prepared all the technical diagrams and pictures. Our thanks to the many colleagues who provided us with impetus for thought and positive feedback in connection with our stroboscopy courses in Berlin. We also thank the publishers for their suggestions. We should be pleased if critical readers would share with us any suggestions for improvement.

Gerhard Boehme (Munich)
Manfred Gross (Berlin)
September 2004

1. Functional anatomy

Many factors are involved in the production of the human voice. The vibration of the vocal folds requires a highly differentiated and precisely co-ordinated series of many individual movements of the larynx. It is important to note that energy is reduced to a minimum while speaking, whereas during singing energy increases. The microstructure of the vocal folds is responsible for a precise series of movements. The vocal tract and neuroanatomy of voice production plays a fundamental role in voice production and biochemical and biophysical factors are also influential.

Microstructure of vocal folds

This consists of:

- the mucosa (epithelium and parts of the lamina propria)
- the vocalis muscle complex (Hirano, 1974).

Lamina propria

The tissue of lamina propria connects to the epithelial layer of the vocal fold. This can be differentiated into three layers:

- *the superficial layer*: this consists of a light connective tissue rich in blood vessels and nerves; the superficial layer of the lamina propria – the subepithelial connective tissue – is analogous to the *Reinke's space*
- *the intermediate layer*: this contains much elastic tissue
- *the deep layer*: consists mainly of collagen fibres, but also contains elastic fibres. (See Figure 1.2)

Using electromicroscopic analysis, Sato (1998) describes how reticular fibres in the superficial and intermediate layer of the lamina propria may be seen. He surmises that the reticular fibres have a key function in maintaining the upright position of the larynx. These fibres also support the viscoelasticity of the vibrating vocal fold tissue.

Vocal cord (vocal ligament) and conus elasticus

These are formed out of the intermediate and deep layer of the lamina propria. The vocal ligament alone forms the upper free edge of the conus elasticus.

M. thyroarytaenoideus (M. vocalis)

Through isometric contraction the muscle can influence the tension of the vocal folds and can also affect vibration ability. The M. vocalis rises as the medial section of the M. thyroarytaenoideus from the inner surface of the anterior surface of the thyroid cartilage and appears in the form of thin fibres on the front surface of the processus vocalis of the arytenoid cartilage.

Muscle spindles occur at the anterior, middle and posterior area in the superior medial quadrants of the M. thyroarytaenoideus. They serve as an elastic receptor and are responsible for a control system in the measurement of the tension and length of the muscle fibres. During differentiated phonation, this function is of great importance. In the *Golgi apparatus*, the muscle spindle is responsible for the biochemical processes (protein synthesis among others) in the vocal folds.

Functional two-layered structure of the vocal folds

The mucosa, the vocal ligament and the M. vocalis all influence the vibration process in different ways, depending on the tension conditions within the vocal folds. The mucosa, consisting of the epithelium and connective tissue, forms a layer which is relatively light and easily moveable. The mucosa is easily identified by stroboscopic means during phonation as a mucosal wave. In contrast, the vocal ligament and the M. vocalis together form a relatively rigid system. Both systems represent the functionally effective two-layered structure of the vocal folds, since the mucosa lies lightly on the rigid ligament-muscle system. This is also referred to as a '*body-cover model*' (Hirano, 1974; Fujimura, 1981) (Figures 1.1, 1.2 and 1.3; Table 1.1).

Anterior and posterior glottis

The *anterior glottis* is a ligamentary intermembranous section, in contrast to the *posterior glottis* which is an intercartilaginous section. The boundary between both sections is the tip of the processus vocalis of the arytenoid cartilage. The actual glottis corresponds to the distance between the anterior commissure and the middle of the

Practical fact

Due to the microstructural features present, the correct term is 'vocal folds'. This is separate from the actual 'vocal cord'. The term 'vocal cord' (Ligamentum vocale) should therefore be avoided whenever one is referring to the entire vocal folds or their mucosa.

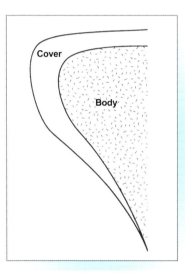

Figure 1.1
Body-cover structure of the vocal folds (coronary section) (Story and Titze, 1995).

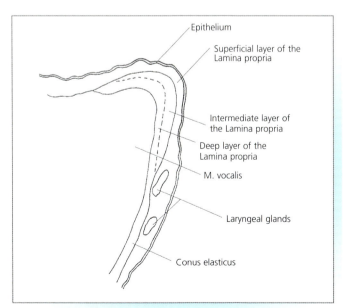

Figure 1.2
Body-cover model of the vocal folds. Histologically there is a five-layer structure, in contrast to a functional two-layer structure (Hirano and Sato, 1995).

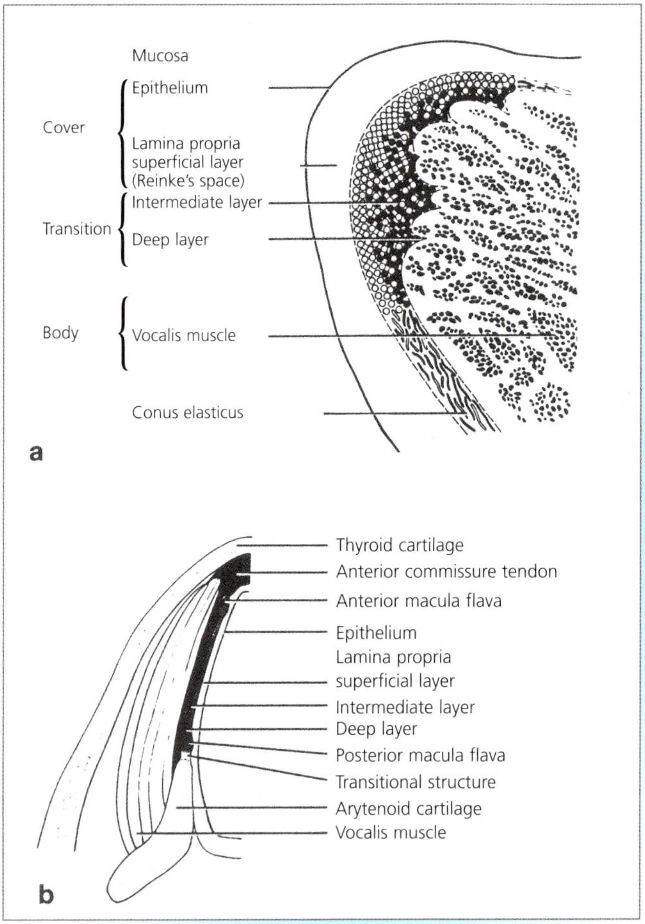

Figure 1.3
Schematic representation of the vocal folds: (a) frontal section, (b) horizontal section (Hirano and Bless, 1993).

Table 1.1 Anatomy, functional morphology and biomechanical features of vocal fold layers					
	Anatomy	**Histological structure**	**Functional morphology**	**Biomechanical stiffness**	**Movement features**
Mucosa	Epithelium	Plate epithelium	Cover	Little	Highest mobility
Mucosa	Lamina propria	Superficial cover layer (= Reinke space), gelatinous	Cover	Little	Highest mobility
Mucosa	Lamina propria	Intermediate layer elastic fibres	Transition	Moderate	Moderate mobility
Mucosa	Lamina propria	Deep layer collagen fibres Ligament.vocale	Transition	Moderate	Moderate mobility
M. vocalis	Muscle	Vocalis fibres of M. thyroarytaenoid.	Body	Strong	Smallest mobility

posterior glottal wall. The designation 'posterior commissure' is incorrect from this perspective. For adults, the ratio of the intermembranous section to the intercartilaginous section is 3:2 (not 2:1) and the ratio of the surface of the intermembranous section to the intercartilaginous section is 2:3 (Hirano, 1991) (see Figure 1.4). Given the modified representation by Friedrich and Lichtenegger (1997) (Figure 1.5) the detailed length dimensions may be calculated.

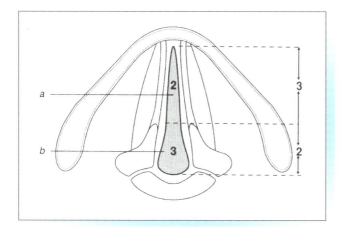

Figure 1.4
Intermembranous and intercartilaginous glottal sections of the glottis:
(a) intermembranous section (anterior glottis);
(b) intercartilaginous section (posterior glottis) (Hirano, 1991).

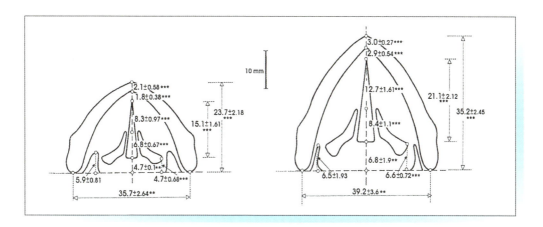

Figure 1.5
Dimensions of the glottal level (adapted from Friedrich and Lichtenegger, 1997).

Average length of vocal folds (in mm)		
	Female	Male
Ligamentary sections	8.3	12.7
Cartilaginous sections	6.8	8.4
Total	15.1	21.1

Subglottal pressure

After a maximal intake of breath on inspiration, pressure amounts to no more than 20 cm H_2O (daPa), which approximately corresponds to the requirements of a very loud speaking voice. Very quiet phonation requires only 3 daPa of subglottal pressure. During singing, subglottal pressure reaches values of 2 to 50 daPa (Proctor, 1980). Subglottal pressure regulates loudness of the voice, while the position of the laryngeal muscles is responsible for the pitch of the voice (Leanderson and Sundberg, 1988).

Glottal output

Performances are based on vocal fold vibrations dependent on time. Vocal fold vibrations occur:

- in 1 second at 200 Hz 200
- in 1 minute at 200 Hz 12,000
- in 30 minutes at 200 Hz 360,000
- in 2 hours at 200 Hz 1,440,000

200 Hz = F_0 (Note: is at the lower end of the range of the fundamental frequency of the female voice)

Primary laryngeal phonation

Primary laryngeal phonation is described as the transfer of glottal signals using indirect examples of laryngeal modelling or clinical investigations. While for the glottal signal only the harmonic tones (overtones) are up to 750 Hz above noise, there are overtones found in the vocal signal which remain above 4 kHz (Klingholz and Arndt, 1988).

Practical fact

Fundamental frequency (F_0) = Number of vibrations of the 'primary laryngeal tones' per second.

2. Physiology

Voice production is based on a precise interaction between subglottal and transglottal forces, which may be partially explained by the myoelastic-aerodynamic theory. In addition to innervation, a balanced proprioceptive system also plays an important role, but it remains unclear which sections exert elastic forces on the vocal folds. Also, the influence of tissue elasticity and viscosity – in addition to the Bernoulli phenomenon of the myoelastic-aerodynamic theory – is not yet clearly known.

Myoelastic-aerodynamic theory

According to the Tonndorf theory (1929) vocal fold vibrations are caused on the one hand by subglottal pressure, and on the other hand by the relation of mass, tension and length of the vocal folds. To explain the mechanics of the vocal fold function, the Bernoulli law of flow for liquids and gasses may be applied and used on the larynx. The air flow passing the glottis not only has the strength to separate the vocal folds, but simultaneously creates the energy to move the folds back together. The glottal area is driven by pressure, suction and perturbation effects.

Biomechanical characteristics of the vocal fold layers

When considered in functional terms, the vocal folds consist of two layers (see above). A 'body-cover model' can be used to explain, on the one hand, mucosa (epithelium and subepithelial tissue) as a flexible system and, on the other hand, the vocal ligament including the M. vocalis as a rigid system. Alternatively, given the vocal fold layers, a division into three may be made (see also Table 1.1). Here even more consideration is given to the stiffness and the phonation movement of the vocal folds.

Biomechanical key phenomena of phonation

The biomechanics of the larynx are not only influenced by anatomical and microanatomical structures. Physical and chemical influences play a far more fundamental role. The following description is based on the findings of I.R. Titze (1998).

- Large molecules (protein fibres and interstitial liquids) determine the material characteristics of vocal folds.
- Material characteristics are measured in terms of density, elasticity and viscosity.
- Elasticity can be directional (along or perpendicular to fibres).
- The material characteristics determine the spread of elasticity waves within the vocal fold tissue.
- Bordering structures (cartilage, tight muscle or air space) determine wave reflections, which lead to standing waves or to normal vibration modes in vocal folds (these resemble formants).
- There is a dense spectrum of normal vibration modes within tissue which results in a large variety of excitations (primarily the stimulation of several vibration modes for periodic air flow impulses on the glottis). Periodic (or aperiodic) air flow impulses serve as a noise source.

Sensory functions of the larynx (proprioceptive system)

Afferent pathways are as important as the efferent pathways for phonation, respiration and the swallowing function. A variety of sensory receptors is spread over the larynx tissue. In addition to chemoreceptors there exists evidence of various mechanoreceptors (see e.g. Cooper and Lawson, 1992).

Proprioceptive sensors are located in the mucosa of the larynx. In addition, receptors are found in muscles (muscle spindles, see above), joints and ligaments. These are located not only in the larynx, but in the lip, tongue and velopharyngeal area. These receptors are involved in the many conscious and unconscious tasks involving laryngeal motor skills. The proprioceptive system, such as depth sensitivity and kinesthetic sensitivity of the larynx, allows control of the actual larynx position within the entire vocal and speech system. During proprioceptional activity, the central nervous system uses all available neural information.

Theoretical larynx models

In biomechanical terms, human vocal folds represent a system of coupled oscillators, which are stimulated to vibrate during phonation.

In order to describe the biomechanics of vocal fold vibrations, theoretical models containing different variables have been developed. A mathematical, computer-simulated, multi-modified model (Figure 2.1) imitates the mass variability contained in the vocal folds in the sense of a body-cover vibration mechanism. It consists of a three-mass larynx model, where the third mass of muscle tissue is simulated. This three-mass larynx model becomes a two-mass model whenever the body mass stiffness becomes extremely high (Story and Titze, 1995).

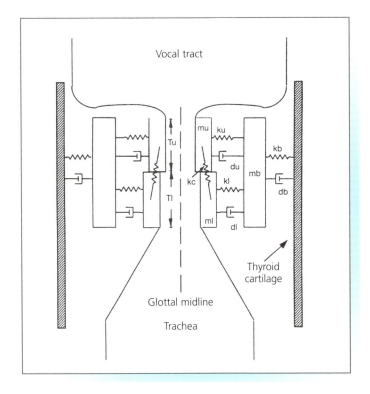

Figure. 2.1
Computer-simulated three-mass model of the larynx (Story and Titze, 1995).

The theoretical results of this larynx model helps intensify our understanding of the physiology of vocal fold vibrations as a stroboscopic image.

Functions of the glottis

The functions of the glottis are amazingly comprehensive and varied. Some important functions are:

- pitch (fundamental frequency of the voice)
- register
- pitch range
- vibrato
- sound pressure level
- projection
- timbre
- voice onset
- precision
- maximum phonation time
- stability
- voice type.

3. Use of optical systems in the glottal area

Optical systems for the analysis of vocal fold vibrations are available in all the varieties also suited for indirect laryngoscopy (Ward et al., 1974; von Stuckrad and Lakatos, 1974, 1975):

1. Rigid laryngoscope with 90° optics
2. Rigid laryngoscope with 70° optics
3. Flexible transnasal endoscope
4. Larynx mirror and microscope with stroboscopic light source
5. Larynx mirror with and without magnification, forehead reflector and stroboscopic light source, adjusted to the forehead reflector.

Rigid endoscopes

The advantage of the rigid endoscope is its good illumination of the larynx. This is especially necessary for video documentation. For daily use, the large areas with deep focus are also very helpful, as sharp images of the larynx and surrounding areas may be produced. If the rigid endoscope contains an optical system with variable magnifying factors (e.g. with two different magnifications), the depth of focus will be somewhat less, but there will be a choice between an overview or a detailed image. A feature of the endoscope's functional principle is that the greater the distance between the endoscope lens and the larynx, the larger the larynx will be shown. An important device for use with the video monitor imaging is the endoscope adapter which contains an additional lens system. This system can be used either for a selected format presentation of the endolarynx or for an overall presentation with additional enlarged sections of the hypopharynx. Although over the past several years a considerable improvement in quality has been achieved, the edges of the image remain more enlarged than the middle sections of the image. This distortion must be taken into consideration during size measurement. The disadvantage of all rigid endoscopes is that during examination condensation may form on the optics from the patient's warm exhaled breath. To prevent this, air insufflators may be used to blow onto the endoscope lens via a feeding tube in the endoscope. Also available is the option of warming the endoscope to body temperature or coating the lens with an anti-fogging material.

An endoscope with high illumination is particularly needed for documentation of vocal fold vibrations. It is therefore important to check the light capacity before purchasing an endoscope, in addition to checking the usual optical and mechanical qualities. Endoscopes with a continuous fibre-optic cable are expensive. There is always a loss of light at the cable junctions. In addition, the cable fibres may become broken through intensive use. Due to the effects of high temperature, carbon particles may eventually accumulate at the cable's junctions. This will lead to a reduction in light strength. The manufacturer may mitigate this effect by polishing the ends of the fibres.

While in Europe 90° optics are preferred for indirect laryngoscopy, a 70° optic is commonly used in the USA. The advantage of a 90° optic is largely the low level of irritation for the patient, thus making the examination easier. A disadvantage cited is the often large distance between the endoscope lens and the larynx and the related lesser-magnified image that can be obtained. Also it is sometimes difficult to adjust the anterior commissure in the case of an overhanging epiglottis, prominent petiolus, or a very strongly developed tongue base. With a 70° optic, the patient's head must be more inclined and the tip of the laryngoscope must be inserted deeper into the hypopharynx. By doing so, the endoscope lens can be guided closer to the larynx and the anterior commissure may be better viewed (see Figure 3.1).

By installing a converter between the endoscope's ocular and camera adapter, it is possible to attain enlargements equivalent to an image from a microscope. The quality of common laryngoscopes by Berci/Ward, Hopkins and by von Stuckrad was analysed by Hahn and Kitzing (1978), Miller and Monnier (1981) and Yanagisawa (1982a, 1982b). Differences were found in the brightness and playback quality with respect to enlargement scale, distortion and image sharpness. The possibility of additional enlargement by sliding an integrated part of the lens system within the optics was achieved by von Stuckrad and Lakatos (1975).

Focusing rings which may be screwed on to common endoscopes are offered as a useful accessory. With the help of these focusing rings it is very easy to focus the endoscope without shaking while holding it with one hand.

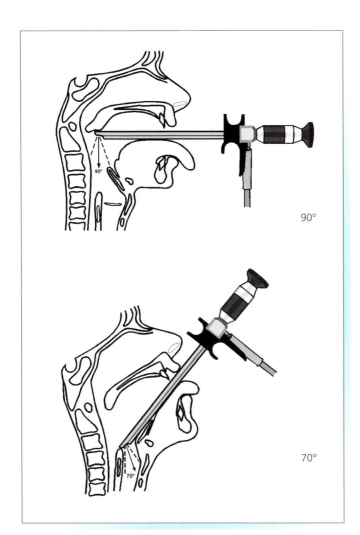

90°

70°

Figure 3.1
Use of 90° and 70° optics.

Flexible endoscopes

Flexible rhino-laryngoscopes are available from various manufacturers in a variety of lengths and diameters, with or without a working channel and with varying light strengths. For connection to the stroboscopic light source there are adapters available for each brand. In practical use with adults and children including video documentation it is necessary to compromise between light strength and endoscope diameter. In practice, imaging using video cameras that are commonly available is not sufficient in the case of endoscope diameter of less than 2 mm.

Using rigid endoscopes for optimal documentation the larynx is shown correctly with the head held precisely upright and the endoscope introduced in the middle line and upright as well. This guarantees that during video recording in normal cases the vocal folds are positioned exactly vertically, and in the case of larynx rotation the image will immediately show the rotation angle. During examinations using a flexible transnasally-inserted endoscope, the image first must be adjusted vertically, if required by readjusting the camera adapter. Predetermined larynx rotations must be taken into consideration.

The advantages of flexible endoscopes are their considerable reduction in gagging reaction and in their use with patients in a lying position or whose mouth opening is inadequate. If an endoscope with strong light is used for imaging vocal fold vibrations, it is normally sufficient to position the tip of the endoscope in the mesopharynx. The weaker the light of the endoscope, the closer the endoscope tip must be guided towards the vocal folds. To prevent irritation whenever swallowing movements elevate the larynx, the endoscope should be pulled back into the epipharynx.

Size measurements

In order to undertake endolarynx size measurements using a rigid endoscope it is necessary to determine the distance between the endoscope lens and the object. From this the magnifying factor results. According to Gross (1988b) the distance between the endoscope lens and the vocal folds may be approximately estimated by measuring the outer distance between the endoscope and the incisura thyroidea and then adding a correction factor of 3.85 mm for women and 4.75 mm for men (Figure 3.2). Several norm values are important to consider when searching for the glottal level from the outer throat (Gurr, 1948; Krmpotic-Nematic et al., 1985). The distance between the incisura thyroidea and the glottal level for women is on average approximately 3.85 mm and for men on average approximately 4.75 mm.

Errors in perspective and distortion

Estimation of size ratio in the larynx may be influenced by image distortion. The resulting changes in the image may be attributed largely to errors in perspective which occur when the optical axis does not stand perpendicular to the projection plane. This in turn is

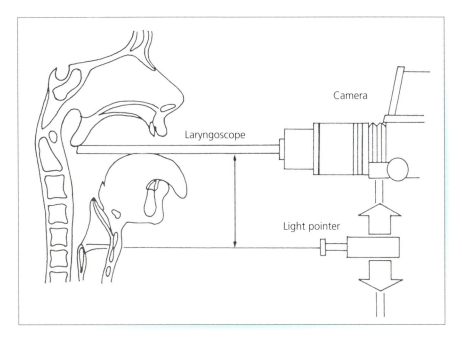

Figure 3.2
Size measurements of the
endolarynx (Gross, 1988).

dependent on the endoscope's position in relation to the larynx, including components determined by the patient's position and the position of the larynx. According to Fleischer, Hess and Ludwigs (1995), when a rigid endoscope is tilted by 40° to the image level, distortions of around 25% occur. This applies to tilting between the endoscope's axis and the vocal fold level as well as to turning of the endoscope's axis. As long as extreme head and endoscope positions are avoided, the authors estimate possible variations between the optical axis and the axis perpendicular to the vocal fold level to be less than 20%, whereby a maximum of 6% distortion occurs. These results were gained empirically and correspond to the calculations of perspective image errors (Lenz, 1990).

Practical fact

During endoscopic vibration analysis, correct patient seating position and correct angling of the endoscope is necessary in order to avoid image distortion.

Flexible endoscopes allow visualization of the entire upper airways and the larynx during speaking and singing. The system is limited by a poor colour representation, by a low image resolution and related coarseness, by a Moiré effect (stripelike effects) and by a considerably greater distortion (fish-eye effect) than in the case of rigid endoscope. As a result, visualization of even small organic lesions is considerably less accurate when using flexible endoscopes (Kost, Eibling and Rosen, 1996).

Microstroboscopy

When examining the larynx with the help of a larynx mirror and a microscope, stroboscopic observation is possible only when a fibre-optic light cable is placed between the stroboscope and the microscope (see also Chapter 5, section 5.6). The advantage of this procedure is good lighting of the larynx and binocular observation. Because of the low depth of focus of the microscope there results an almost fixed magnifying factor between the object in question and the resulting image. Thus microscope recordings are particularly suited for quantitative analysis using size measurement. The drawback of this technique is believed to be a mirrored representation. In addition, this method requires good co-operation by the patient and also a certain amount of practice on the part of the examiner. Selecting various magnifications it is possible to achieve overview images as well as closely enlarged detailed imagery.

Laryngostroboscopic examinations using a larynx mirror with or without magnification, whereby stroboscopic light is aimed on the larynx using a forehead reflector, are rarely practised today. The advantage of this technique is the low discomfort for the patient. The disadvantage is, in contrast, the limited lighting of the endolarynx, with mirror-reversed imagery.

4. Auditory voice assessment and vibration analysis of the vocal folds

Examiners use a very large number of criteria to describe the voice, depending on the variety of vocal qualities. Within the literature, various category systems are used: GRBAS according to Hirano (1981); RBH according to Wendler et al. (1996); GRBASI according to the guidelines of the Belgian Study Group on Voice Disorders (Heyning et al., 1996).

Furthermore, distinctions are made between an auditory voice assessment of the voice onset (breathy, soft, hard), voice placement (frontal, pharyngeal, backward) and the voice offset (soft, firm, hard).

The results of the auditive voice assessment and vocal fold vibration analysis are closely related. Table 4.1 underlines the interrelation of the above-mentioned RBH classification (R – Roughness, B – Breathiness, H – Hoarseness) in relation to stroboscopic and acoustic findings.

Table 4.1 Interrelation between stroboscopic, auditory and acoustic findings		
Stroboscopic	*Auditory*	*Acoustic*
All variations	Hoarse	Additional noise components
Irregularity	Rough	Change in the fundamental frequency
Incomplete glottal closure	Breathy	High frequency noise induced by tubulent air flow
Source: adapted from Wendler et al. (1996).		

The limits of explaining the relation between an auditory voice sound and stroboscopic findings are quickly reached, for example when it is attempted to compare a 'lumpy' voice sound (brought about through changes in the vocal tract) or a pressed voice function in relation to vibration analysis of the vocal folds.

5. Stroboscopy

5.1 Preliminary remarks

The clinical value of stroboscopy is undisputed and well-proven in the case of organic and functional dysphonia. Over the course of recent years this has been demonstrated in an exemplary manner in the following cases.

- Woo et al. (1991) evaluated 146 dysphonic patients. With the aid of stroboscopy 15 patients (= 10%) experienced a modification of their laryngologic diagnosis (without videostroboscopy). Additional significant information was gained for 27.2 % of the dysphonic patients evaluated with videostroboscopy.
- With the help of videostroboscopy, Sataloff et al. (1991) found that 18% of 377 patients had been diagnosed incorrectly.
- According to Remacle (1996), of 732 patients 13% required a correction of diagnosis after videostroboscopy was used. In 68% of the cases the diagnosis was groundbreaking. In 17% of the cases the initial diagnosis was modified to functional dysphonia after videostroboscopic findings; in 20% of patients a vocal fold nodule diagnosis was made; in 23% of cases there was a Reinke's oedema, while granulomas were found in 17%.
- Cantarella (1998) analysed the value of videostroboscopy for laryngological diagnose for 456 patients suffering from hoarseness (with the exception of larynxparalysis and neurological diseases). In 18% (82 patients) a modification of the diagnosis could be made with the aid of videostroboscopy.

Although the use of stroboscopy has considerable advantages, the examiner should nevertheless be aware of many limitations involved (see Table 5.1).

Fields of application for stroboscopy

The diagnostic and differential diagnostic possibilities of stroboscopy are extremely comprehensive. Possibilities differ widely for organic and functional voice disorders.

Organic voice disorders
- Local findings of the glottis
- Neurological reasons
- Pre- and post-operative diagnostics for phonosurgical operations.

Table 5.1 Advantages and disadvantages of stroboscopy
Advantages of stroboscopy   Good picture quality   Moving images   Summary of vibration process simultaneously for the entire glottis
Disadvantages of stroboscopy   True-to-nature imagery only with strictly periodic vibrations   No continuous series of images   Subjective evaluation   Quantitative evaluation only with additional video or film recording   Quantitative evaluation is time consuming   Difficult evaluation during short phonation

Functional voice disorders
- Exclusion of minimal organic changes in the glottis
- Quantitative evaluation of different vibration phases with consideration of loudness, subglottal air pressure, glottis configuration, vocal fold tissue structure and tone of the glottis muscles.

Sensitivity and specificity of stroboscopy

Organic and functional voice disorders are evaluated differently with the aid of laryngostroboscopy. Fundamentally, organic voice disorders provide more certain results than functional voice disorders. Thus the criteria with respect to sensitivity and specificity vary greatly for organic and functional voice disorders. In the case of organic dysphonia there is a high level of sensitivity, yet limited specificity. In the case of functional dysphonia there is a low level of sensitivity, yet no specificity (Wendler, 1997) where sensitivity is the probability of recognizing an ill patient and specificity is the probability of recognizing a healthy individual.

Training programme for the evaluation of stroboscopic findings

1. Poburka and Bless (1998) recommend a computer-supported training programme for individual stroboscopic evaluation. *Computer-aided instruction (CAI)* is based on visual approximation of various stroboscopic parameters involved in video imagery. After four to five hours of training, examiners without previous knowledge are able to obtain good understanding of various stroboscopic options (including evaluation criteria).

2. An additional training programme is *LVES (Laryngeal Videoendostroboscopy)* (Irby and Hooper, 1997). A general voice knowledge test is recommended for the evaluation of the glottis function. Using a multiple-choice technique, questions are asked using video clips, for instance:

The patient in this video has

(a) an increased mucosal wave and a posterior opening of glottis?

(b) a decreased mucosal wave and an hourglass-shaped glottis?

(c) a normal mucosal wave and a posterior glottis closure?

(d) normal mucosal wave and an hourglass-shaped glottis closure?

The test contains 30 further questions. The training programme is supplemented by additional tests.

5.2   Historical overview

References in medical history to the subject of stroboscopy provide surprising insights into technical, laryngological and phoniatric presentation. The chronological progress of development helps to improve our understanding of the numerous possibilities in the application of video laryngostroboscopy.

For those interested, the individual works, book contributions and monographs of authors such as Weiss (1932), Sovák (1945a, 1945b), Panconcelli-Calzia (1957), Schönhärl (1960), Leden (1961) and Hirano and Bless (1993) provide further information on the historical development of 'illusory viewing', that is, stroboscopy.

If the human eye did not react in such a languid manner there would be no such thing as stroboscopy. The English physician and inventor of the periodic electrical current breaker, Peter Mark Roget (1779–1869), was one of the first to investigate what had been known even hundreds of years previously: it is possible to create the optical illusion of continuous movement by using what is in reality a series of individual images.

1829

Joseph Antoine Ferdinand Plateau (1801–83), a Belgian professor, taught physics at the University of Ghent. In one of his 1836 works he described the laws of 'stroboscopic effect'. Already in 1832 he set up a device to test his ideas which he called a *phenakistiscope* or *phantoscope*. It consisted of a circular-shaped disc with pictures along the edge which was rotated quickly and reflected into a mirror. Through slits in the disc edge it was possible to observe the mirrored images as they turned. Plateau attempted this with 16 pictures per second – a recording frequency which was later used in silent films.

1832/33

Simon Ritter von Stampfer (1792–1864), a professor of mathematics in Vienna and a measurement specialist, described the stroboscopic principle in new terms. In contrast to Plateau, von Stampfer worked with two discs which were attached exactly opposite each other on an axle. One disc held pictures, the other was cut with slits. He called the device a *stroboscope* or *circular turning viewer*. Both the phenakistiscope and the stroboscope had the disadvantage that the pictures were distorted into an angular form since their return distance was further at the edge of the disc than at the axis. This disadvantage was eliminated by the Englishman William George Horne (1786–1837), with his *zoetrope*, also known as the *life turner* or *wonder drum*. Using this device, one could look through a slit to view a series of pictures located opposite on the inside of a drum which turned on a vertical axis. The paper strips with the picture series could be replaced.

1852

E. Harless was the first to observe the mechanism of voice production of the larynx using cadavers.

1866

A. Töpler noted the possibility that stroboscopy might also be suitable for investigations of human phonation:

> The blowed cords of a natural or artificial glottis very clearly reveal a change in form during the various phases of vibration. It cannot be doubted that with the help of a mirror in the throat and intensive lighting that the vibroscope [Töpler's name for the stroboscope] would also be suited for the physiological study on living glottis during phonation (Panconcelli-Calzia, 1957).

1877

The Frenchman Emile Reynaud improved upon Horne's zoetrope or wonder drum with his *praxinoscope*. A series of flat mirrors attached to a second inner drum intermittently reflected the continuously circling pictures attached to an outer drum(Figure 5.1).

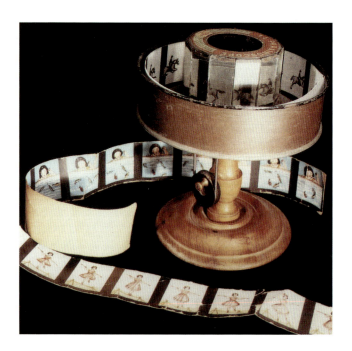

Figure 5.1

A stroboscope for the observation of the motion process with a picture sequence placed into a hollow drum. The drum is lit from the open side; the picture change is achieved by using a mirror prism attached to, and rotating with, the drum; by fixing one's vision on to a certain position in the mirror, one picture at a time is viewed; when a sufficiently fast rotation is achieved, an impression of movement appears. (Naturwissenschaft und Technik, 1991).

1878

In the mid-1870s Eadweard Muybridge built a giant set in California in which a horse 'filmed itself'. The shutters of 24 photographic cameras connected in series were released when a horse galloped by and tripped trigger wires. With the 24 photos Muybridge was able to prove that there were certain times when none of the horse's hooves touched the ground while galloping (Figure 5.2).

1878/1895

Max Joseph Oertel (1835–98) (Figure 5.3), employed as an internist and laryngologist in Munich, introduced stroboscopy to the field of human laryngology. In a preliminary report in 1878, Professor Oertel described a laryngostroboscopic examination in detail. The *perforated disc stroboscope* (Figure 5.4) that he used was perforated in three rows.

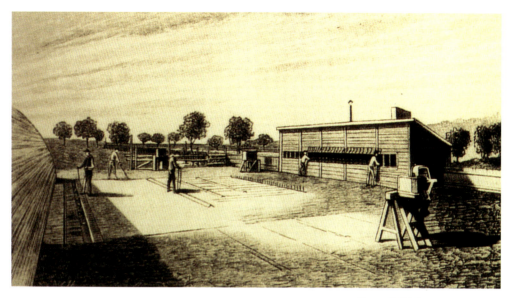

Figure 5.2 (a)
Muybridge's giant set for obtaining his photographs of a galloping horse.

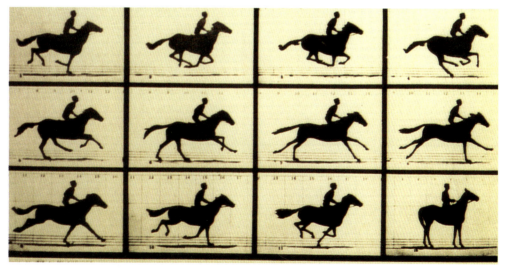

Figure 5.2 (b)
Muybridge's 24 photos of a galloping horse (Naturwissenschaft und Technik, 1991).

1898
Albert Musehold (1854–1919) made the first photographic images of the vocal folds.

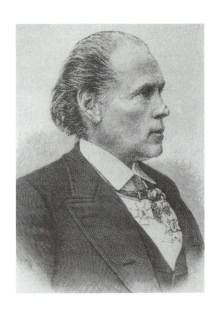

Figure 5.3
In 1895 Max Joseph Oertel (1835–98) introduced human stroboscopic testing for the evaluation of vocal fold vibrations.

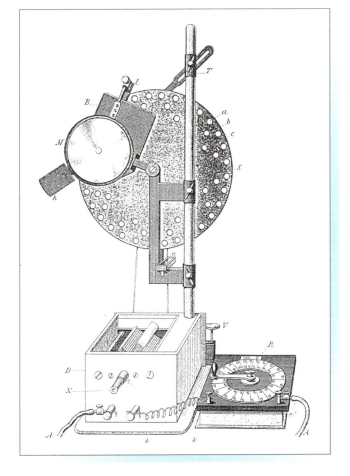

Figure 5.4
Early mechanical stroboscopes used a perforation in front of a constant light source to pulse the light; according to Oertel (1895).

1921
Miroslav Seeman (1892–1975) introduced stroboscopic methods into voice pathology.

1932
Leo A. Kallen and H.S. Polin developed the first electronic stroboscope. Instead of using rotating discs they used a light flash which test patients controlled themselves using a microphone located at the larynx or in front of the mouth. This replaced the perforated disc stroboscope (Kallen and Polin, 1937).

1945
M. Sovák (Prague) published a two-volume monograph on laryngo-stroboscopy.

1957
Bernhard Vallancien was the first to describe 'Stroboscopie et télévision' and thus may be considered the father of video-laryngostroboscopy.

1960
Elimar Schönhärl published a monograph with the title 'Die Stroboskopie in der praktischen Laryngologie' (Stroboscopy in Practical Laryngology) which is in a large part still valid today.

1977
Volker Barth expanded the diagnostic possibilities using stroboscopy with endoscopes.

1978
Gerhard Kittel established the actual technique of videostroboscopy with his 'Endoscopic-Micro-TV-Colour Stroboscopy'.

1979
Y. Yoshida developed videostroboscopy using a direct recording of a stroboscopic glottal image, whereby a camera is directly connected to the optic system.

1993
Minoru Hirano and Diane M. Bless published the important monography 'Videostroboscopic Examination of the Larynx'.

In the long development of laryngology, the technique was first applied mainly in Europe for scientific and clinical purposes. Over the course of the past few decades the technique has spread worldwide. Along with further development, considerable developments in research have taken place in Europe, North America, and Japan. At the start of the twenty-first century stroboscopy has gained importance around the globe and has become an irreplaceable, routine technique in laryngology and phoniatrics.

5.3 Basic principle of stroboscopy

For a better understanding of laryngostroboscopy, a basic discussion on the biophysics of vocal fold vibrations is necessary.

With the help of indirect laryngoscopy using normal, constant lighting, only rough vocal fold adduction and abduction adjustment movements can be recognized on the larynx in connection with phonation and respiration. These movements are active processes which are controlled by nerve and muscle activities. In contrast, vocal fold movements occur with considerably smaller deflection and in a passive manner through the exhalation of air during phonation.

The vocal folds vibrate at such a high frequency that their movements cannot be recorded during an indirect laryngoscopy or an endoscopy via rigid endoscopelaryngoscopy without additional apparatus. Without such apparatus there is a visual impression of motionless vocal folds in a phonation position, or possibly the impression of unclear vibrations which are not further differentiated. However, with the aid of stroboscopy, vibrations may be observed.

Talbot's Law

Stroboscopy is based on Talbot's Law. According to this law, the time resolution of the human eye is clearly limited. Every visual impression is retained on the retina for about 0.2 seconds. Faster movements thus cannot be discriminated. A more rapid process (more than five images per second) using clear and distinct pictures, gives an impression of continuous motion in which several various movement phases are experienced as overlapping each other.

Still and moving images

The principle of stroboscopy takes the physiological features of the human eye into consideration. With the help of a series of flashes the individual phases of a movement process can be exposed. The vibration phases in between are not illuminated and thus not visible. The human eye fuses together the movement phases that are illuminated. Given favourable conditions, this technique can be used to help us understand vocal fold movement as they appear to the eye. Given unfavourable conditions, the examiner may receive the illusion of an unusual movement process of the vocal folds.

If the same vibration phase is illuminated during a period of vibration, an impression of a still image will occur (Figure 5.5). The series of flashes is controlled by a generator so that the same vibration phase of each of a consecutive series of vibrations may be illuminated precisely.

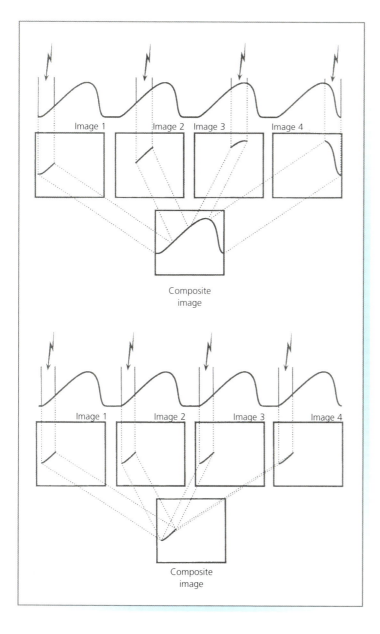

Figure 5.5
Still and moving. Above: a moving image is obtained through the illumination of consecutive phases. Below: A still image is obtained through multi-illumination of the same vibration phase.

If the series of flashes is set up so that consecutive movement phases of various vibratory cycles for a periodic vibration are illuminated, then the impression will be that of a moving process – that is, a moving image (Figure 5.5). In order to differentiate individual phases, the length of flash must be very short. With the help of modern Xenon flash lamps, a flash length of less than a thousandth of a second may be attained.

By the use of monochromatic or multi-colour light diodes (LEDs) attached to the tip of the laryngoscope, Hess and Ludwigs (2000a, 2000b) presented a very cost-effective and uncomplicated electronic variation for illumination with continuous and flash lighting. Another current development used for stroboscopy involves continuous halogen lighting interrupted by a shutter.

To observe different vibration phases using still images, the examiner has the option of slightly changing the flash series using a foot-operated switch. Using this method, an observation of the phase process may be made in 'slow motion'. Should the examiner wish to observe a moving image proceeding forwards, then the flash frequency must be reduced permanently lower than the vibration frequency. Normally here the distance between the light flashes is selected to be 0.75 Hz below the basic frequency of the vocal fold vibrations. For a more rapid movement process, a frequency 1.5 Hz less than the vocal fold frequency is chosen.

Microphone control

To control the flash generator, the vocal fold vibration frequency must be determined by the means of a frequency analyser and a microphone – this is known as microphone control. This involves

Practical fact

A *still image* is obtained when the light flash always hits the same phase of a vocal fold vibration. A *moving image* is when the light flashes illuminate various phase sections during consecutive periods. The appearance of a still image of different phases may be attained using a *foot switch* to create minor changes in the flash frequency.

an audible pitch at the fundamental voice frequency. For men, this is normally calculated using the speaking voice with a basic frequency of 98 Hz (G) to 131 Hz (C) and for women 196 Hz (G) to 262 Hz (C_1). If necessary, stroboscopy will be used beyond these values for lower or higher frequencies. This applies for vibration analysis below modal fry (low frequencies) or for singers above the speaking voice level (high frequencies within the musical voice range). Microphone control using an airborne vibration microphone may occur in three ways:

- the airborne vibration microphone is mounted on a magnifying endoscope
- an airborne vibration microphone can be hand held or mounted on a tripod
- a physical vibration microphone is fastened to the collar microphone in a prelaryngeal percutaneous manner.

Delta-t generator

The flash frequency is set approximately by using the microphone or tone generator control. With the help of a delta-t generator, the flash frequency may be varied by a small amount. If the delta-t is small, it will take longer to complete an entire cycle. If a larger delta-t is chosen (adjustable by using the foot switch on some equipment), a rapid series of individual pictures will result and/or fewer pictures per cycle are presented.

Tone generator control

An additional option involves a fixed setting of the flashlight frequency, requiring the patient to phonate at the frequency at which the flashlights are triggered. That is, tone generator control occurs. It is also possible for the examiner to phonate into the microphone for voice frequency analysis and attain a flash frequency via the microphone control (see also above). This last technique may be applied particularly in cases of diplophonia, during which the examiner imitates one of the two tones and thus clearly controls the flash frequency. However, this technique is also very prone to disturbance. If the patient is not in a position to phonate at a given frequency, the examiner must adjust the flash series to the fundamental frequency of the patient during tone generator control.

Practical fact

Triggering the stroboscopic flash
- Microphone control
- Automatic fundamental frequency analysis of the microphone signal

Tone generator control

- Patient phonates at a given pitch
- Physician adapts the tone generator to the patient's pitch

Practical fact

Use of tone generator control
- for extending a tone length which is too short
- to improve synchronization
- where automatic fundamental frequency is distorted
- where microphone signal is too weak

Vibration phases

High-speed films of vocal fold vibrations from the 1940s had already shown that in normal cases a closing movement follows the opening movement of a vocal fold. This is followed by a closed phase in which both vocal folds are in contact (in the modal fry). Correspondingly, the phases are described as opening, closing, and closed phases. The opening and closing phases are together referred to as the open phase, because air can move through the glottis during this phase. The sum of the open and closed phases amount to one vibratory cycle (see Figure 5.6).

Glottic configurations, subglottal pressure and the consistency of the vocal folds (including muscle tone) all have an effect on the vibrations of vocal folds. Since subglottal pressure and vocal fold consistency are practically non-determinable during vibration analysis, vocal fold vibrations can only be partially determined.

Vibration forms with varying levels of loudness

There is a clear connection between loudness levels and vibration amplitudes. During soft phonation the glottis opens in a considerably

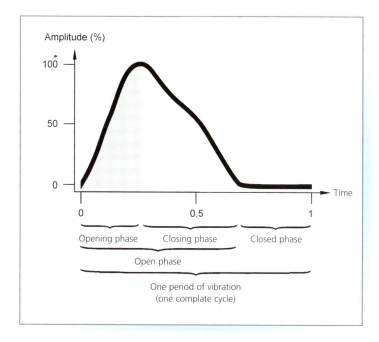

Figure 5.6
Vibration amplitude in various phases of a vibratory cycle.

more extended manner and should it even slightly touch the vocal fold the closed phase will be lengthened with increase loudness. Simultaneously the amplitudes are larger. According to Timcke et al. (1958) the glottis always remains open even during the most soft phonation (see Figure 5.7).

Vibration forms independent of the voice register

See section 5.4.

Inferior laryngoscopy

In an experimental study, Salimbeni and Alajmo (1985) investigated the stroboscopic process of subglottal mucosa movements in ten

Practical fact

Phases of vocal fold vibrations
Open phase

- Opening phase
- Closing phase
- Closed phase

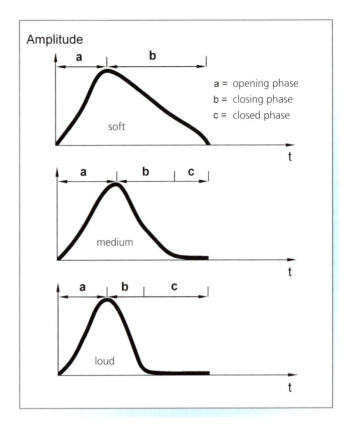

Figure 5.7

Vibration behaviour during soft, medium and loud voices. With soft voices the glottis is open during the entire vibratory cycle. The glottis closes completely and for a longer interval as loudness levels increase (Timcke et al., 1958).

tracheotomized patients prior to a laryngectomy. Upward movement was found in the mucosa, caused by the subglottal pressure and this movement proceeded to the edge of the vocal fold. A forward and sideways movement of the vocal fold edge was thereby caused. Inferior laryngoscopy confirms the aerodynamic – myoelastic phonation theory.

Synchronized stroboscopic images with video image sequencing

During video recording of stroboscopic images it must be remembered that the European PAL system records 25 frames per second while the NTSC system found in the USA records 30 frames per second. Each frame consists of two fields displayed in two passes. To guarantee an even level of light for all pictures, it is necessary to include additional synchronization between the light flashes and image frequency. This is the only way to ensure that a light flash is triggered for each frame. (Figures 5.8 and 5.9).

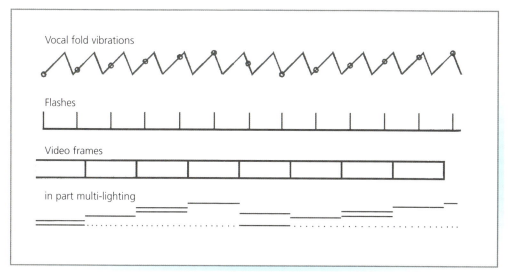

Figure 5.8
Video recording of stroboscopic images (multi-lighting during videostroboscopy). Through high frequency of the vocal fold vibrations, part multi-lighting will occur for each full video image. (Ludwigs, Orglmeister, Hess und Gross, 1996).

Figure 5.9
Video recording of stroboscopic images with additional synchronization. Despite a higher frequency of vocal fold vibrations, multi-lighting is avoided through the use of additional synchronization at video frame frequencies (European PAL system 25 Hz, US NTSC system 30 Hz). (Ludwigs, Orglmeister Hess und Gross, 1996).

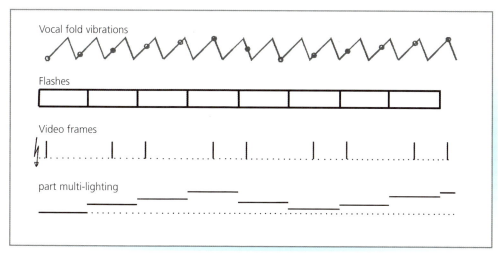

5.4   Normal stroboscopic vibratory pattern

The normal physiological *vibratory pattern* of vocal folds involves three movements (Figure 5.10):

- a horizontal movement from median to lateral
- a vertical vibration that swings from caudal to cranial
- wavelike movements of median vocal fold surfaces with opening of the glottis from the caudal to cranial direction.

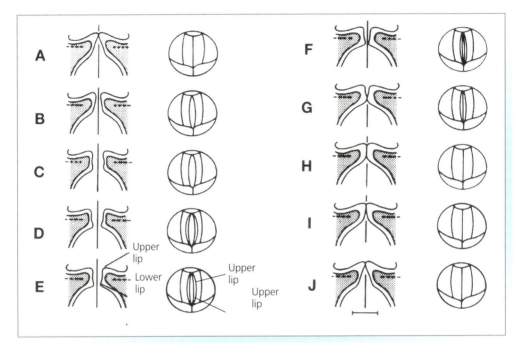

Figure 5.10
Schematic illustration of normal stroboscopic movement process
Left column: frontal level; right column: top view. (Hirano and Bless, 1993, modified from Schönhärl, 1960).

Normal vocal fold vibrations are characterized by regular, even-sided movements from a middle amplitude, complete closed phase and clear mucosa shifting (Figure 5.11). In the lower frequencies the vocal folds vibrate along their entire length and width, and show clear movements in the mucosa in the mediolateral and lateromedial direction in the form of a mucosal wave. With increasing pitch, the amplitudes and mucosal waves decrease. In contrast, amplitudes increase with increasing loudness, and the mucosal wave becomes more prominent. In the upper levels of the physiological range the vocal folds are tight.

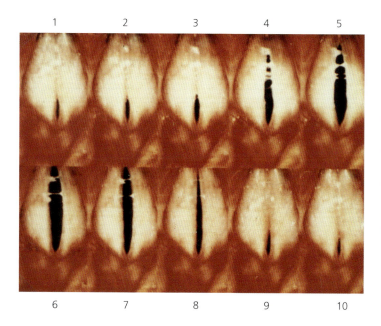

Figure 5.11
Stroboscopic image of a normal vocal fold vibration. Top: 1 closing phase, 2–5 opening phases; below: 6–9 closing phases; 10 closed phases. (Courtesy of Kay Elemetnics).

Stroboscopy and voice register

In order to describe the normal stroboscopic vibration process, it is first necessary to be familiar with the various vibratory patterns for individual voice registers. Fundamentally a distinction can be made between the following:

- vocal fry, pulse
- modal fry, and
- head register, falsetto (men) and whistle register (women and children).

A differentiated laryngostroboscopic analysis may be seen in Table 5.2. A schematic illustration of vibratory patterns comes from Hirano and Bless (1993) (Figure 5.12). According to these authors, the voice register is best evaluated at the modal fry level, since here the vocal folds vibrate in their full range and reveal a large amplitude.

Table 5.2 Stroboscopic analysis of vocal register	
Vocal fry	Aperiodical vibrations, large amplitude, complete glottis closing, supraglottal constriction
Modal fry	Vibrations in entire range, large amplitude, prominent mucosal wave, complete glottal closure
Head register	Periodic vibrations, very small amplitude, incomplete glottal closure

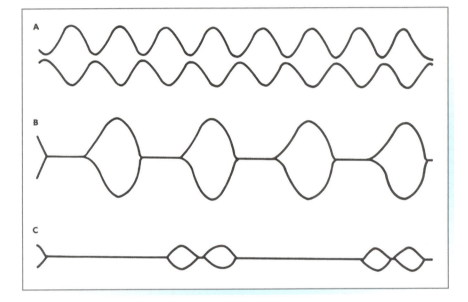

Figure 5.12
Schematic illustration of stroboscopic finding of the voice register. A = Head register, B = Modal fry, C = Vocal fry (Hirano and Bless, 1993).

5.5 Evaluation criteria

Stroboscopy allows for an oriented and differentiated observation of vocal fold vibrations during phonation. Stroboscopy without acoustic pressure level measurements and evaluation of fundamental frequency, only provides a general impression of the vocal cord vibration. It also provides information when an infiltrating process occurs. Thus this procedure is valuable as an additional test. In combination with rigid and fibre laryngoscopy and the inclusion of video technology using digital methods the technique has proven itself well during routine examinations. For differential analysis and scientific analysis it is necessary to include the acoustic pressure level and frequency for qualitative and quantitative prognosis.

Basic considerations during videostroboscopy

- Videostroboscopy is always just a part of a multi-dimensional vocal diagnostic.
- The videostroboscopic image is dependent on the acoustic pressure level dB(A) and the phonatoric fundamental frequency (f_0) in Hz.
- The evaluation of videostroboscopic findings is largely dependent on the experience of the examiner.

Stroboscopic evaluation criteria

- The analysis of glottis configuration on the basis of video-endoscopy via a rigid endoscope (without videostroboscopy) is an indirect technique for determining glottis geometry. The key focus is on the pre- and post-operative comparisons of surgery to improve the voice. Here it is necessary to be able to recognize possible influences on the results of qualitative and quantitative stroboscopic analysis.
- Qualitative videostroboscopic evaluation criteria include features such as the glottal closure, amplitude, symmetry, periodicity, regularity, mucosal wave, phonatory immobility and supraglottal constriction .
- Quantitative videostroboscopic evaluation criteria refer to a differentiated examination of each phase and phase process. The individual phases many be counted and compared, thus allowing time-related behaviour to be determined.

5.5.1 Determination of glottis configuration

Stroboscopic vocal fold vibration processes are dependent on the geometry of the glottis configuration determined through laryngologic assessment. The results must be included in the qualitative and quantitative stroboscopic evaluation criteria. Equally important factors are derived from the viscosity and elasticity of the larynx tissue.

Thus, within the framework of an overall stroboscopic analysis, it is necessary to discuss the geometry of glottis configuration during phonation and respiration, as this serves in the preparation of subsequent qualitative and quantitative stroboscopic analysis of vibration processes.

Technique

There are several techniques for the analysis of glottis configuration. They are based in part on digital image processing, whereby video images are used to measure laryngoscopic findings via a rigid endoscope. This involves determination of angles and glottis lumen calculations (in pixels).

Method according to Woodson (1993) In connection with laryngeal paralysis, videolaryngoscopic findings in two dimensions are investigated with the help of angle determination (Figure 5.13).

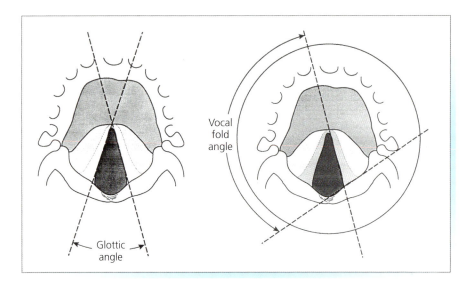

Figure 5.13

Glottis during inspiration. Above left: anterior glottis angle is determined (also during excavation or bulging) between the anterior commissure and the Proc. vocalis. Right: Anterior vocal fold angle is determined between the anterior (membraneous) and the posterior section of the vocal fold (Woodson, 1993).

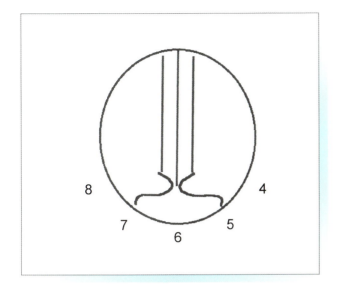

Figure 5.14
Glottis position (GP). Median position of the vocal fold Position 6. Respiratory movement right up to 8, left up to 4 (Pahn and Dahl, 1995).

Method according to Kleinsasser et al. (1994) The use of a laryngometer (combination of a slide gauge with a Storz-Hopkins lens) allows a scaled determination of theglottis surface in square millimetres.

Method according to Pahn and Dahl (1995, 1996) Computer-supported data processing of laryngoscopic findings of the glottis function is proposed. Outside the vocal fold vibration process, information on the glottis function is gleaned through the following features: 1. Glottis position (GP) (Figure 5.14), 2. glissando reaction (GLISS), 3. Respiratory movement of the arytenoid cartilage (RMA), 4. Respiratory movement of the vocal folds (RMV), 5. Glottis (G), 6. Symmetry of the Ary-Wrisberg-Santorini cartilage (AWS).

The results are given in number form and build on the clock code for recording symmetry and respiratory motility as well as division of the glottis into thirds for a description of a possible incomplete glottal closure. The data for each side are provided separately. Median positioning of the glottis occurs when there is a laryngoscope value of 12 for the posterior commissure and a value of 6 for the anterior. A normal respiratory movement of the arytenoid cartilage is sufficient when the right value is up to 10 and the left up to 2. The glottis is divided into thirds: posterior, medial and anterior, and given split formation the lumen is assessed for each side for each third. Computer analysis allows a schematic graphical reconstruction of the visual laryngoscopic image result on the monitor and allows classification of vocal status and of vocal function tests.

Method according to Inagi et al. (1997, 1998) Glottal measurement for one-sided vocal fold paralysis (1997) and for thyroplastic conditions (Type 1) (1998) is undertaken direct from the monitor using a videostroboscopic classification with the help of pixel determination. Measurement of the glottal width, length and angle is recommended.

Method according to the computer program, Dr. Speech (1998) With the aid of special software the glottis angle is determined. A graphical representation with raster division is used.

Over the past few years more information has been obtained on mapping the glottis surface through pixel counting of digitalized videostroboscopic frames.

Conclusions

Determination of glottis configuration prior to stroboscopic examination is valuable in patients with:

- vocal fold paralysis
- larynx rotation
- limited movement of the arytenoid joint, e.g. due to tumour infiltration or rheumatoid changes
- N. laryngeus superior paralysis and
- before and after a thyroplasty.

Furthermore with the aid of the methods described above, a precise glottis configuration analysis for differentiation between flaccid and taut vocal fold paralysis may be obtained.

5.5.2 Qualitative stroboscopic evaluation criteria

Before a qualitative stroboscopic evaluation can take place, a precise analysis of the glottis configuration is required. All abnormalities should be integrated into the overall plan for stroboscopic vocal fold analysis.

Numerous authors have written in detail about stroboscopic evaluation criteria and recommended some testing schemes (Table 5.3). Building on these investigations, Table 5.4 (page 42) contains an independent summary of stroboscopic evaluation criteria of vocal fold vibrations and disorders.

Table 5.3 Stroboscopic evaluation criteria

Recommendations from:	
Kitzing (1985)	Remacle (1996)
Bless, Hirano, Feder (1987)	Ott (1997)
Schuerenberg (1990)	Boehme (1997)
Woo et al. (1991)	Stemple, Gerdemann, Kelehner (1998)
Hirano, Bless (1993)	Dejonckere et al. (1998)
Hoefler (1995)	Postma et al. (1998)
Bless, Hicks (1996)	Cornut, Bouchayer (1999a)
Wendler et al. (1996)	Poburka (1999)
Friedrich (1996)	Boehme, Gross (2001)
Colton and Casper (1996)	

A short form of the stroboscopic evaluation criteria contained in Table 5.4 is suitable for documentation of findings in daily practice (Table 5.5, page 43).

Eight evaluation criteria should be observed during stroboscopic analysis. These form the main part of stroboscopic assessment. The eight criteria will be described in detail in the following section.

Eight stroboscopic evaluation criteria
1. Glottal closure
The glottal closure is an important criterion for the qualitative analysis of vocal fold vibrations. In addition to normal glottal closure, there are six other schematic variations of differences in incomplete glottal closure, as seen in Figure 5.15, page 44.

Besides a complete glottal closure, the following also may occur:

- a posterior incomplete glottal closure
- a incomplete glottal closure from front to back
- an hourglass-shaped glottis
- an arch-shaped incomplete glottal closure
- an anterior incomplete glottal closure
- an irregular glottal closure.

With the exception of a small or a narrow incomplete glottal closure in the posterior third, all other forms lead to a breathy voice. Therefore an incomplete glottal closure should be sought in the closed phase with the aid of stroboscopic analysis.

Table 5.4 Qualitative analysis of vocal fold vibrations: evaluation questionnaire according to Boehme and Gross (2001)

1. Glottal closure

complete (normal)	posterior incomplete glottal closure	incomplete from front to back	hourglass-shaped	arch-shaped	arch-shaped and post triangle	anterior incomplete glottal closure	irregular	other

2. Amplitude

	normal	increased	decreased	missing
Right				
Left				

3. Symmetry (of phases)

	normal	slight phase shift	distinct phase shift
(right phase/ left phase)			

4. Periodicity

4. Periodicity (continous succession of periods)	Periodic	aperiodic (frequency change periods)

5. Regularity

5. Regularity	normal vibration form	irregular	longitudinal

6. Mucosal wave

	normal	increased	decreased	missing
Right				
Left				

7. Phonatory immobility

7. Phonatory immobility	not present	partial	total
Right			
Left			

8. Supraglottal constriction

Not present	anterior-posterior	false vocal folds: right/left/both	other

Table 5.5 Qualitative stroboscopic evaluation criteria and functional disorders

Evaluation criteria	Functional disorders
1. **Glottal closure**	see Figure 5.15
2. **Amplitude/glottis width** - during intensity increase: increased - during intensity reduction: decreased - during increasing pitch: decreased - description: small, medium, large	- increased - decreased - fluctuations in amplitude (irregularities) in the form of blurred contours within still image.
3. **Symmetry** - right amplitude /left amplitude - opening and closing movements occur on both sides simultaneously and symmetrically	- asymmetric - phase shift between right and left vocal fold
4. **Periodicity** - no additional changes in frequency	- aperiodicity, frequency change periods
5. **Regularity**	irregularity
6. **Mucosa wave** - Wave-formed (medial) shifting of the mucosa in contrast to the toned M. vocalis	- reduced or missing
7. **Phonatory immobility** - amplitudes and mucosal wave during phonation apparent	- Amplitudes with mucosal waves are not apparent
8. **Supraglottal constriction (additional finding)** - **pathological**	- Contact between false vocal folds - Contact between epiglottis and arytnoid cartilage

Recommendations

- Regular examination at a specific frequency (e.g. 131 Hz = C_1, 262 Hz = C_2) as monitor insert
- Regular examination at certain sound pressure levels (e.g. 60 dB) as monitor insert.

A narrow posterior division in the stroboscopic movement image does not necessarily need to be evaluated as a pathological finding. In contrast there may be an appearance of an hourglass-shaped glottis as the result of one or two-sided findings (cysts, polyps, vocal fold nodules) on the free edge of the vocal fold.

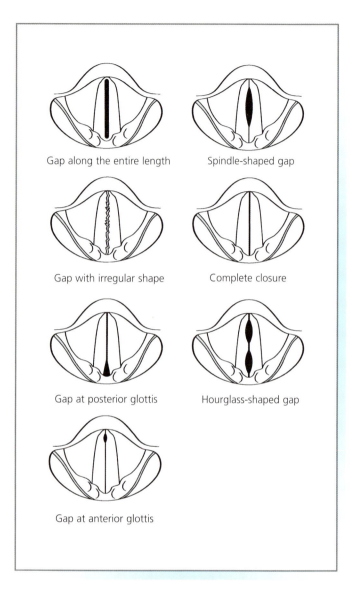

Figure 5.15
Various possibilities of an
incomplete glottal closure.

Gap along the entire length

Spindle-shaped gap

Gap with irregular shape

Complete closure

Gap at posterior glottis

Hourglass-shaped gap

Gap at anterior glottis

2. Amplitude

This evaluation criterion involves the medio-lateral deflection of each individual vocal fold, that is, *each vocal fold is evaluated from the left and the right in isolation*. Here we may find either a normal, extended, shortened or missing amplitude. When the voice intensity increases, the amplitude does as well. In the case of a pathological increase of stiffness in the vocal fold, amplitude will decrease. The separate analysis of the right and left amplitudes thus may lead to a glottis image asymmetry given a one-sided amplitude change.

If both amplitudes are observed simultaneously, one may see the glottis width, which is the maximum deflection of both vocal folds together in a medio-lateral direction at the respective vibration phase. The tone of the glottis is of predominant importance. It should be considered independently of the amplitude, particularly in functional voice disorders.

3. Symmetry

Normally all movements of the *two vocal folds* occur symmetrically. That is, the vibration phases of the right vocal fold begin at exactly the same time as on the left vocal fold. Normally the amplitudes for both sides are the same. If the vibration phases of both vocal folds are shifted against each other, this is referred to as a phase shift or phase difference. The amount of the phase shift is described as a percentage or in degrees, whereby a period of 100% corresponds to 360°. A phase shift should be regarded as a pathological finding, although it rarely occurs in those with healthy voices.

4. Periodicity

The process involved in vocal fold vibrations normally takes place in periods. A periodicity occurs when the vocal fold vibrations follow each other at the same interval. An *aperiodicity* is the so-called *period of frequency change*. This may be a sign of a functional disorder and appears as a missing frame in the stroboscopic pattern. A slight tremolo in the voice may also be detectable as a period of frequency change.

5. Regularity

Regular forms of vibration occur when the movement occurs as illustrated in Figure 5.10 (page 34).

'Irregular' is understood to be:

- longitudinal vibrations in the vocal fold area
- up and down movements of the vocal folds (for instance the paralytic vocal fold presents with movements like a flag flapping in the wind)
- in the case of an hourglass-shaped glottis, either the posterior or anterior area may be affected only; there may also be varying speeds between the posterior and anterior areas.

6. Mucosal wave

A mucosal wave involves a wave-shaped shift of the mucosa (epithelium and Lamina propria) in contrast to the tonalized M. vocalis (see also see Figure 5.10, Schœnhaerl, 1960).

The mucosal wave can be normal, strengthened, decreased or eliminated.

7. Phonatory immobility

A phonatory immobility is an important symptom for organic vocal disorders; for example, in the case of carcinoma of the vocal fold, it is characterized by a complete loss of amplitude and mucosal wave. Independent of pitch and loudness, no vibrations are recognized on the affected vocal fold. Usually, a one-sided phonatory immobility takes place. Reversibility within a short period of time indicates a benign affliction of the vocal fold.

Phonatory immobility is a serious indication of limited movement ability of the muscosa. It occurs, for example, in cases of closure due to scarring between the mucosa and M. vocalis, during infectious alterations involving deeper-located tissue layers, or during infiltrative processes

8. Supraglottal constriction

A supraglottal constriction occurs during excessive levels of muscle activity in the anterior-posterior and/or latero-medial direction.

- An anterior-posterior symptom (epiglottis near the arytenoid region) may result in an apparent shortening of the vocal fold; in addition, the following may occur:
- The one-or two-sided false vocal folds during phonation can shift in the median direction; in an extreme case both false vocal folds come into contact with each other during phonation so that a vocal fold stroboscopy is no longer possible.

5.5.3 Quantitative stroboscopic analysis

The aim of a quantitative analysis of stroboscopic findings is the exact description of individual vocal fold vibration phases. Our knowledge of vibratory behaviour is based largely on high-speed kinematographical assessment by Timcke (1956), Timcke, Leden and Moore (1958, 1959) and Leden, Moore and Timcke (1960) as well as a number of other authors such as Duncker and Schlosshauer (1961) and Arndt (1994).

The quantitative analysis of vocal fold vibrations is difficult. Only very few authors have attempted to evaluate vocal fold vibrations systematically. (e.g. Woo, 1996).

Opening, closing and closed phase
The basis of quantitative analysis of vocal fold vibrations is knowledge of the opening and closing movements of the vocal folds during phonation. A vibratory cycle may be divided into two phases: the open phase during which the glottis is open, and the closed phase in which both vocal folds normally make contact with each other. In the open phase it is again possible to differentiate between two contrasting movements: the opening movement and the closing movement. The corresponding phases are thus referred to as the opening and closing phases. A complete vibratory cycle is made up of an opening and closing phase (the same as an open phase) and closed phases (see also Figure 5.6, page 31).

The vocal fold vibrations are not only considerably dependent on pitch, loudness, form and consistency of the vocal folds, but are also dependent on subglottal pressure. During stroboscopic diagnostics it is not practically possible simultaneously to check this subglottal pressure.

The open phases become smaller with increased frequency. After this the opening function of the glottis is no longer sinus shaped, but triangular shaped.

As well as the time relation between the open phase and the total period, there are other important factors for quantitative vibration analysis. A prime factor is the amplitude and possible existing phase shifting between the left and right vocal folds. The vibration amplitude of a vocal fold is the maximal deflection in the medio-lateral direction. In contrast, the vibration width relates mainly to the entire glottis. Correspondingly, the maximal distance between both vocal folds during medio-lateral vibration movements is defined as

Practical fact

Vocal fold vibrations are influenced by various factors which cannot be accurately measured during stroboscopy. Thus the interpretation of findings is difficult and prone to error.

the vibration width. Determination of vibration amplitudes in millimetres assumes that the enlargement factor (e.g. the vocal fold image on the video monitor) and the original size of the object are known. During endoscopic stroboscopy this is possible only with much effort (Gross, 1989). More practical is the calculation of symmetry quotients in which the maximal amplitudes of the right and left vocal folds are set in relation to each other. In an ideal case there is a symmetry quotient of 1. Over the course of years a series of additional quotients has been defined: their advantage is that an absolute determination of phase durations is not required.

Quotients
- *Vibratory cycles* (total period) = opening phase + closing phase + closed phase.

The terms 'vibratory cycles' and 'total periods' are equivalent.

- *Opening quotient* = opening phase / total period.

Using the opening quotient, the relation of the opening phase to the entire vibratory cycle is described. With an increase in voice loudness, the opening quotient normally becomes smaller.

- *Speed quotient* = opening phase / closing phase.

This quotient describes the relation between lateral movement and medial movement.

If the voice volume increases, the closing phase becomes shorter and the vocal folds move more quickly from a lateral position to a medial position.

- *Closed quotient* = closed phase / total period

Practical fact

Vibratory cycle (P)
- Duration of a vibratory cycle (with opening phase, closing phase, closed phase)
- Opening phase + closing phase + closed phase
- $P = 1/F_0$

The closed quotient is complementary to the open quotient; it is added together with the open quotient to amount to a value of 1.

In assessing a vibratory cycle, a check is made whether the various vibration phases occur simultaneously in the right and left vocal folds, or whether they are shifted against each other. To quantify a phase shift, a single frame technique is used during stroboscopy. A practical method is to count the number of images from the beginning of the closed phase of the right vocal fold, until the closed phase of the left vocal fold begins. This number is compared to the number which completes a whole vibratory cycle. Phase shifting is normally expressed as a percentage or in degrees. One cycle amounts to 100% or 360°.

The quantitative analysis of vocal fold vibration is based on observation of individual vibration phases. Of most importance is the relationship between the opening and closing phases. While analytic techniques such as electroglottography, kymography and high-speed recording are used to determine the actual length of the different phases, video documentation may be used during stroboscopy to determine the number of individual frames contained during each vibration phase. The number of individual frames per phase can be compared in the form of quotients. The open quotient has proved itself to be especially informative in determining the ratio between the open phase and an entire vibratory cycle. The closed quotient (the relation between the closed phase and the entire vibratory cycle) is complementary to the open quotient and thus provides no additional information. In concrete terms, the determination of open quotients with the aid of videostroboscopy involves the technique of counting single individual frames: counting how many individual frames are contained in the open phase and within an entire period. The relation between these two numbers is equivalent to the open quotient. In order to evaluate a complete cycle, it is recommended that you always begin at the start of a closed phase, as this is easy to determine. In an ideal case, the closed phase begins with the first complete glottal closure. If the glottal closure is incomplete or is completely missing, then under some conditions the closed phase is reduced to a minimal duration; the closure merely represents the turning point between the opening and closing movement during a deflection at a maximal medial direction. According to kymographic examinations made by Gross (1988), the open quotient is normally between 0.5 and 0.8 for average loudness and fundamental frequency of the speaking voice.

In the case of hyperfunctional dysphonia the open quotient is a value of <0.5; in the case of a hypofunctional dysphonia the value is > 0.8. Additional laryngoscopic and/or stroboscopic indications of hyperfunctional dysphonia are: reduction of the anterior-posterior distance of the supraglottis, protrusion of the petiolus, hyperadduction in the arytenoidal area (possibly with the so-called overlapping phenomenon), hyperadduction of the vocal folds, prominent a false vocal fold, a shortened vibration amplitude, a lengthened glottal closure, mucous strands between both vocal folds at the transition of the anterior and middle vocal fold third, as well as a marginal discrete reddening on both sides of the medial vocal fold edge; this may be interpreted as working hyperemia.

5.6   Examination techniques

Basically it is possible to divide stroboscopic techniques into the following:

- endostroboscopy and
- microstroboscopy.

Both techniques may be practised in the form of videostroboscopy. Generally, endostroboscopy is more widely used. In contrast, microstroboscopy is applied more in cases of phonosurgery and for differential diagnostics, e.g. between cysts and polyps.

Stroboscopy via rigid endoscope

Rigid endoscopy (Barth, 1977) expanded the diagnostic possibilities for stroboscopy, as it is very helpful for patients with a poorly visible endolarynx.

(a) This allows a stroboscopic evaluation of the anterior commissure, especially in the case of hyperfunctional dysphonia with a dorsal-positioned epiglottis. Even in cases of strong gag reflex, rigid endoscopy allows easier evaluation of vocal folds.
(b) Rigid endoscopy allows observation of vocal folds with

Practical fact

For endostroboscopic diagnostics, rigid endoscopes and fibre endoscopes are used.

magnification up to six times. This makes detailed diagnostics of vibrations during phonation considerably easier, e.g. during a mucosal wave.

(c) Furthermore, better lighting of the endolarynx is an added advantage.

Laryngostroboscopy via fibre endoscope

Observations of vocal fold vibrations with the help of a flexible endoscope (transnasal) and stroboscope allows the fibre optics to move as close to the vocal folds as possible. This technique is preferred for patients whose strong gag reflex makes an indirect laryngoscopy or a rigid endoscopy impossible. This examination has the advantage that the physiological speaking process is affected very slightly. However, the image quality is not as good compared to rigid endoscopy.

Microstroboscopy

The combination of stroboscopic techniques with the magnification possibilities of an operation microscope is described by the term microstroboscopy (McKelvie et al., 1970; Pascher et al., 1971; Seidner et al., 1972). Advantages are the magnification of vocal fold images as well as binocular viewing. *Telemicrostroboscopy* consists of microscopic magnification of vocal folds while using the advantage of the stroboscopic effect and the application of a TV monitor. The details of mucosal movements (e.g. mucosal waves) are especially easy to recognize using microstroboscopy, so that this technique may be used partially during *indirect microsurgery on vocal folds* (Wendler et al., 1996).

Videostroboscopy

Using his rigid micro TV colour stroboscope, Kittel (1978) provided evidence on the excellent application possibilities of the common and routine technique of videostroboscopy. While performing the test, the examiner views the monitor instead of looking into the patient's mouth or through a camera. For clinical routine diagnostics, video-stroboscopy has become widespread.

Why use videostroboscopy?

1. There are considerable advantages when dealing with patients: since examinations are recorded, the recordings may be used to help patients gain a better understanding of the findings. Also, the type and range of laryngeal function and various therapeutic measures may be explained to the patient.

2. The fundamental frequency (f_0) in Hertz and the sound pressure level in dB during phonation may be added to the currently-running video frames.
3. Stroboscopic video documentation of laryngological findings is easy and cost-effective.
4. The technique is well suited to demonstration purposes when teaching.
5. With the aid of a video printer it is possible to print a black and white or colour picture of the findings immediately for the medical files, which would be useful for those involved in further treatment of the patient.

Seating position of the examiner

A right-handed examiner should sit opposite the patient to the right; a left-handed examiner should sit opposite the patient to the left. For right-handers, the video system should be positioned to the right of the patient.

Rigid stroboscopic examination techniques

The left index finger should not rest on the upper lip, but should lie as a support under the rigid endoscope. In this way the endoscope is properly fixed.

90° and 70° lens optics

For indirect routine laryngoscopy and stroboscopy of the larynx, rigid 90° and 70° endoscopes may be used. While the device must be guided horizontally into the mesopharynx when using 90° lens optics, the endoscope must be tilted further in the caudal direction when using a 70° optics lens. At the same time, the 70° optic lens system will be guided more closely towards the larynx, which leads to increased magnification. When a 70° endoscope is successfully placed, the examiner can obtain a clearer view of anterior commissure.

Topical anaesthesia during stroboscopic examination

During *stroboscopy via rigid endoscopes* a routine anaesthesia of the throat with Lidocain spray is not necessary. In any case, a tendency to gag may possibly impede the undisturbed observation of the stroboscopic vibration process of the vocal folds. In this case, a mucosal anaesthesia of the rear pharynx is necessary.

An anaesthetic of the nasal mucosa during a *transnasal fibrelaryngo-stroboscopy* is not mandatory but more comfortable for the patient.

Leder et al. (1997) proved this using a double blind study. According to this investigation, influence of transnasal examination is negligible – with or without local anaesthesia of the nasal mucosa – on the results of stroboscopic vocal fold diagnostics.

Multifunctional stroboscopic systems

During routine stroboscopic examination, it is necessary to optimize functional diagnostics. The use of image insertion techniques for relevant data shown on the video monitor is indispensable, in addition to the LCD display and orientated stroboscopy.

The following test data should be visible on the monitor with the aid of image insertion techniques:

- patient data and date during phonation with continuous registration
- fundamental frequency (f_0) in Hertz
- sound pressure level in dB.

Possible additional test data of a jitter and shimmer registration serve to supplement the monitor display as mentioned above. This also applies to the insertion of continuous electroglottograms (EGG).

Practical fact

Only through use of insertion techniques can a differentiated interpretation and comparison with previous findings be made during videostroboscopy. Additionally, the insertion technique allows easy documentation.

Examination process during videostroboscopy

For everyday practice the following videostroboscopic method is recommended:

1. Anamnesis

2. Otorhinolaryngological assessment

3. Rigid laryngoscopy
   if needed: Mucosal anaesthesia of the pharynx
                                     90° and additionally 70° lens

90° rigid laryngoscopy: position patient correctly
upright posture
head straight ahead
horizontal view

70° rigid laryngoscopy: position patient correctly
cervical and thoracic vertebral
column tilted forwards

4. Flexible transnasal fibre endoscopy
if needed, nasal mucosal anesthesia

5. Preparation of video recording, that is, presentation of the following data will be displayed on the monitor in synchronization with the stroboscopic examination

Surname, First Name
Date
Relevant test data
Fundamental frequency of the voice (Hz)
Sound pressure level in dB
Jitter, shimmer (if needed)
Phase (eventually)

6. Videorecorder in stand-by mode.

7. Assessment of the fundamental frequency of the voice and pitch range.

For patients involved in speaking professions, there should be at least a stroboscopic assessment of the pitch range, corresponding to the fundamental frequency of the voice during voice load. The normal fundamental frequency of the speaking voice is between G and C_1 for men. For stroboscopic assessment this means:

G = 98Hz
A = 110 Hz
H = 123 Hz
C_1 = 131Hz

for women between G_1 and C_2. For stroboscopic assessment this means:

G_1 = 196 Hz
A_1 = 220 Hz

$H_1 = 247$ Hz
$C_2 = 262$ Hz

8. Stroboscopy with microphone positioning

   Moving image with air conduction microphone (hand held or fastened to the rigid endoscope)
   Moving image with microphone held to the neck with collar clip
   Still image if needed
   Clarify phase shift with glottal closure

9. If needed, a stroboscopic examination is made of the musical pitch range. This is especially necessary in cases of glottis carcinoma or when dealing with singers. First, a stroboscopic examination is done for the corresponding pitch range. This is followed by a stroboscopic examination for all frequency ranges

10. Tone generator control.

This examination is necessary in cases of:

   – a phonation length which is too short
   – non-musical patients.

Here two methods are possible: The patient is asked to phonate and the examiner adjusts the stroboscope's flash series precisely to the patient's fundamental frequency. This is done by regulating the pitch of the tone generator manually.

The examiner sets a pitch range using the tone generator at which the patient is likely to be able to phonate easily. The patient is then asked to phonate in the suggested pitch range.

Practical fact

A stroboscopic examination made at a head register may lead to inadequate results in the vibration process of the vocal folds. Basically, laryngostroboscopy should follow in the pitch range (for men between 98 and 131 Hz, for women between 196 and 262 Hz). The singing voice (up to 1000 Hz) may be evaluated in addition if needed.

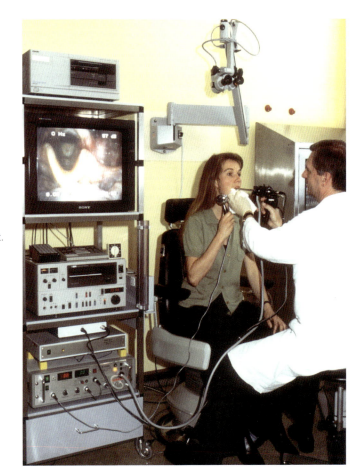

Figure 5.16
Laryngostroboscopic assessment.

5.7 Organic voice disorders

Stroboscopy is an essential method of assessing numerous acute and chronic laryngologic disorders. Its differentiated application requires comprehensive basic knowledge of the morphological and clinical progress of disorders – especially in the glottal area. Indeed, the use of stroboscopy for individual disorders varies greatly. The following description should serve to outline the importance of various clinical applications of videostroboscopy for various vocal fold disorders.

5.7.1 Laryngitis (including reflux laryngitis)

Stroboscopic examination allows us to recognize the grade of *acute laryngitis*. Findings should correlate to vocal fold vibrations and may be taken as a prognostic indication. Acute laryngitis affects the superficial layer of the lamina propria and is thus localized in the mucosal area. The various findings – dependent on the degree of severity – may possibly include the cover of the vocal fold and may even result in a phonatoric immobility.

Chronic laryngitis in the form of hyperplastic alteration is amenable to stroboscopic assessment. Here phonatoric immobility must be excluded which may indicate carcinoma in situ or early progress of vocal fold carcinoma (see also Section 5.7.9). Apart from this, chronic laryngitis is limited to the mucosa and reveals varying stroboscopic symptoms which depend on the degree of severity (Figure 5.17 a–d).

Reflux laryngitis with granuloma

A reflux laryngitis is not uncommon and may be evaluated as outlined above using stroboscopy to trace clinical progress. A step-by-step normalization of various stroboscopic assessment criteria using medical therapy is thus of real benefit in voice diagnostics and therapy.

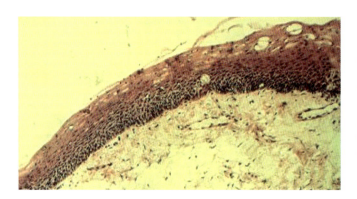

Figure 5.17a
Chronic catarrhal laryngitis: Histology: showing the early stages of hyperkeratosis with koilocyts. (After Behrendt: Histological archive of the ENT. University Hospital, Leipzig).

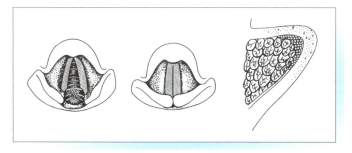

Figure 5.17b
Superficial layer of thhe lamina propria. (Hirand and Bless, 1993).

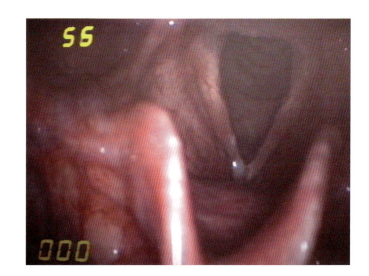

Figure 5.17c
Video endoscopic findings in respiration position

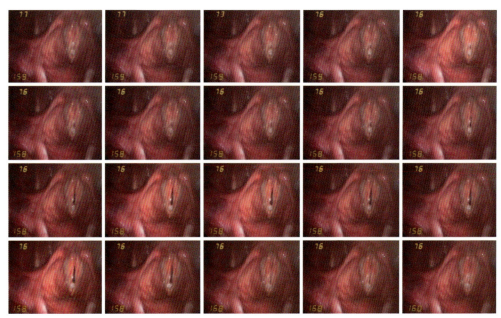

Figure 5.17d
Stroboscopic video sequence.
Glottal closure: complete
Amplitude: reduced
Symmetry: present
Periodicity: periodic
Regularity: normal waveform
Mucosal wave: reduced
Phonatoric immobility: not present
Supraglottic constriction: not
    present

Figures 5.18a and b underline the value of stroboscopic diagnostics for patients with laryngo-pharyngeal reflux and granuloma in the processus vocalis area, including hyperplasia in the interarytenoid region. After a two-week protone pump inhibitor treatment, laryngologic and stroboscopic analysis reveals that the granuloma is no longer present (Figures 5.19a and b).

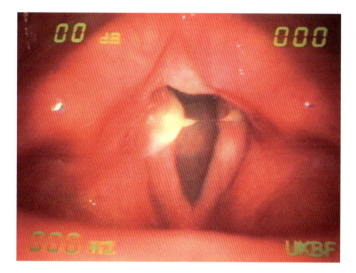

Figure 5.18a
Laryngo-pharyngeal reflux with granuloma on the right processus vocalis and hyperplasia within the interarytaenoid region (before treatment). Young male patient, 30 years.

Video laryngoscopy: during respiration granuloma on the right processus vocalis with mucous fibres towards the opposite side (see also Figure 5.18b).

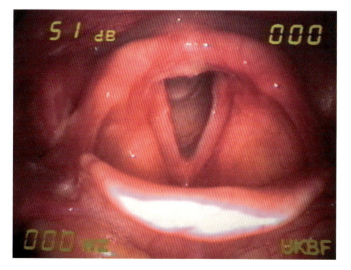

Figure 5.18b
Status of laryngo-pharyngeal reflux with granuloma formation in the right area of the processus vocalis after two weeks' treatment with proton pump inhibitor medication. Young male patient, 30 years.

Video laryngoscopy: In the respiration and phonation position no granuloma is present. Hyperplasia improved in the interarytaenoid region (see also Figure 5.19b).

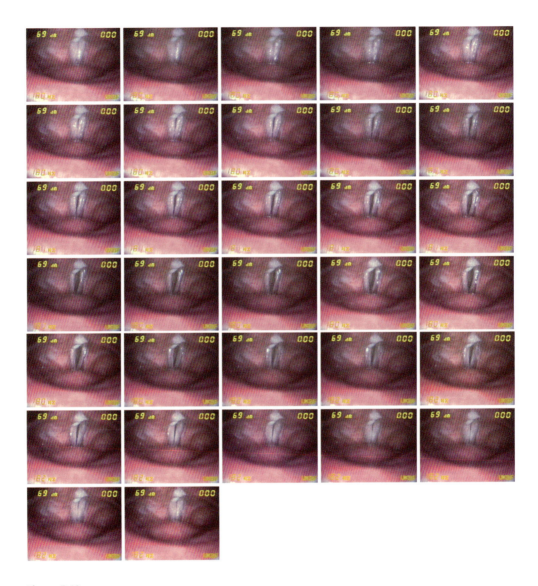

Figure 5.19a

Laryngo-pharyngeal reflux with granuloma at the right arytenoid cartilage and hyperplasia of the interarytenoid region (before treatment) in a 30 years old male patient A.

Video stroboscopy (Picture b):

Glottal closure: complete

Symmetry: present

Amplitude: wide

Periodicity: regular

Mucosal wave: not noticeable

Phonatoric immobility: not present

Vertical vibration direction: not pathological

Supraglottic constriction: not pathological

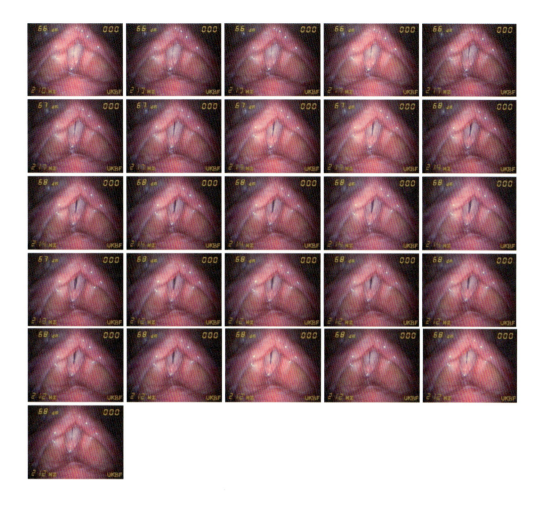

Figure 5.19b
Patient A two weeks after
medication with Omeprazol.
Video stroboscopy:
Glottal closure: incomplete along
  the entire length
Symmetry: asymmetric
Amplitude: right medium large.
  Left small (head register)
Periodicity: present
Mucosal wave: not pathological
  (head register)
Phonatoric immobility: not present
Vertical vibration direction: not
  pathological
Supraglottic constriction: not
  pathological

5.7.2 Vocal fold bleeding, varicose veins and telangiectasia

Vocal fold bleeding

Vocal fold bleeding, mainly in evidence on one side, is located within the superficial layer of the lamina propria (Figure 5.20 a–c). From a clinical viewpoint, microvascular lesions (varicose veins or telangiectasia, see below) may be isolated by macroscopic means. Hirano and Bless (1993) aptly describe vocal fold bleeding as 'subepithelial bleeding of the vocal folds'.

Stroboscopic evaluation is essential within the framework of a clinical diagnosis. An asymmetry results due to one-sided vocal fold bleeding. Depending on the extent of the problem, the affected side reveals an increase in cover stiffness including a slight increase in the cover substance mass. Amplitude and mucosal waves on the affected side are smaller than on the unaffected side (Hirano and Bless, 1993).

Figure 5.20a
Subepithelial bleeding in the left vocal fold.
Diagram (after Hirano and Bless, 1993). The superficial layer of the lamina propria (cover) is affected.

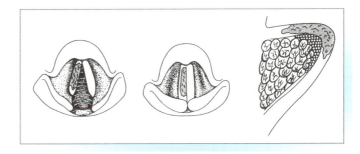

Figure 5.20b
Video laryngoscopic findings in respiration position.

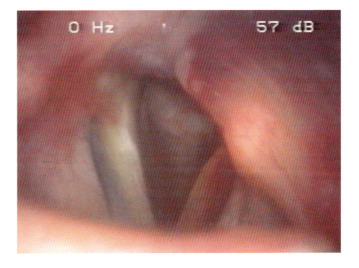

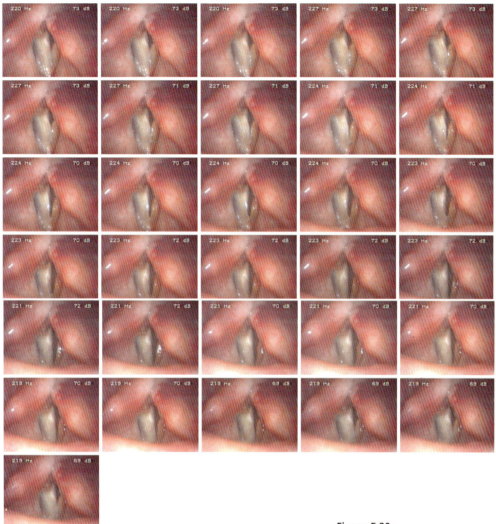

Figure 5.20c
Stroboscopic video sequence:
Glottal closure: posterior gap
Amplitude: right normal, left
  reduced
Symmetry: phase shift
Periodicity: periodic
Regularity: normal vibration pattern
Mucosal wave: right normal, left
  reduced
Phonatoric immobility: not present
Supraglottic constriction: not
  pathological.

Spiegel et al. (1996) describe a comparison of stroboscopic findings at the initial stage and during check-ups (Table 5.6). Among other things, the checks revealed that an improvement of the mucosal waves was detected in all patients. A partial normalization of stroboscopic findings took place.

Table 5.6 Comparative stroboscopic findings in patients with initial vocal fold bleeding and during follow-up (Spiegel et al., 1996)		
Stroboscopic findings	Initial (n = 23)	Follow-up (n = 23)
Decreased amplitude	20	15
Decreased waveform	19	12
Incomplete glottal closure	12	4
Vocal fold mass	7	7
Varicosity	4	6
Normal examination	0	7

Conclusion

Patients displayed multiple signs of a vocal fold dysfunction. Seven patients demonstrating residual decreases in amplitude and/or waveform had only minimal increased stiffness.

Varicose veins and telangiectasia

Microvascular lesions such as varicose veins and telangiectasia should be distinguished from hemorrhagic polyps, nodules, cysts, granuloma and larger arteriovenous deformations. (Postma et al., 1998). A stroboscopic analysis is essential prior to phonosurgical measures. For instance, during a mucosal wave assessment a better localization of varicose veins and/or telangiectasia may be obtained.

5.7.3 Vocal fold nodules

Vocal fold nodules normally appear bilaterally and symmetrically and are located in the superficial layer of the lamina propria. (Figure 5.21 a–d) Schönhärl (1960) described the differences between soft and hard vocal fold nodules in detail. In connection with hard nodules he mentions the hourglass-shaped glottis.

A detailed description of qualitative stroboscopic assessment criteria of vocal fold nodules is found in Hirano and Bless (1993):

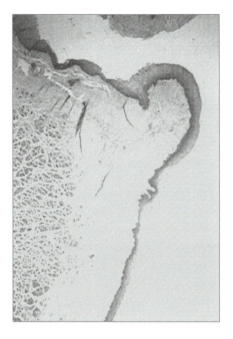

Figure 5.21a
Vocal fold nodules
Histology (after Hirano in
Sataloff, 1997); in this example
the epithelium and the
superficial layer of the lamina
propria is affected; it contains
collagenous fibres and an
oedema.

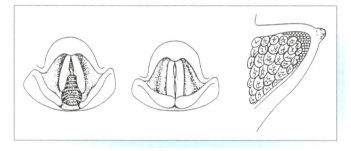

Figure 5.21b
Diagrammatic representation of
Figure 5.21a (Hirano and Bless,
1993); the superficial layer of the
lamina propria (cover) is affected.

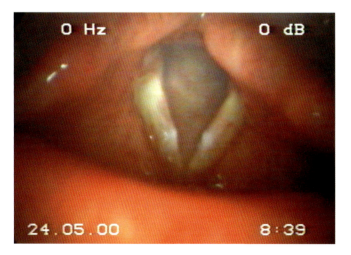

Figure 5.21c
Video laryngoscopic findings in
respiration position.

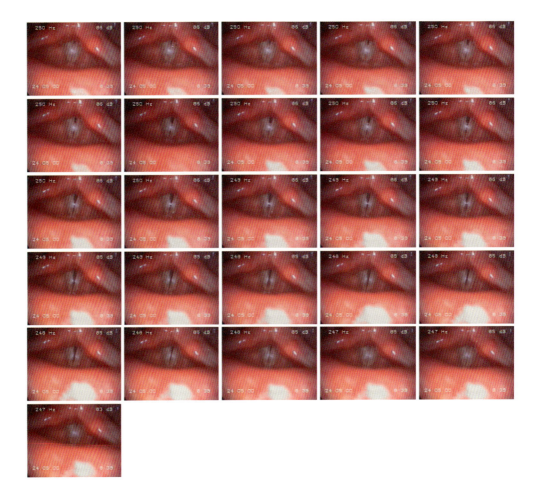

Figure 5.21d

Vocal fold nodules; stroboscopic video sequence:

Glottal closure: posterior gap

Amplitude: reduced

Symmetry: present

Periodicity: periodic

Regularity: normal vibration pattern

Mucosal wave: reduced

Phonatoric immobility: not present

Supraglottic constriction: present.

To some extent, a glottal closure is not reached. A symmetry of both vocal fold vibrations is nearly present. The stiffness of the cover varies depending on the histological features. That is, vocal fold stiffness increases in the case of fibrous nodules, and decreases given oedematous nodules. Overall the cover mass increases somewhat. The body remains untouched. There is no increase of stiffness and mass. The vocal fold nodules also disturb the vibratory movements of the contra-lateral vocal fold. Stroboscopic findings should include an hourglass-shaped glottis with a maximal closure. The amplitude is reduced on the right and left. The mucosal wave in that region is not present if the vocal fold nodules are fibrous and solid; that is, the mucosal wave isolates the nodule area. In contrast, the mucosal wave may often be seen in cases of soft nodules. *Basically, the histological character of vocal fold nodules can be expanded to a limited extent through a precise analysis of mucosal waves.*

Due to these qualitative stroboscopic assessment criteria, the differentiation between oedematous and hard (fibrous) vocal fold nodules is made easier. Together with clinical findings and after careful checks, it can be decided whether a conservative or operative treatment is most promising method.

According to Gross (1998a), a videostroboscopic differential diagnosis of hard and soft vocal fold nodules is not always possible, and transitions must be considered. Thereafter, hard (fibrous) vocal fold nodules may lie in a very superficial position and provide evidence of a mucosal wave. These findings may be proved through postoperative histological evaluations, in which there is evidence that vocal fold nodules may become fibrous.

5.7.4 Vocal fold cysts

According to Arens et al. (1997), 58.2% of 416 laryngeal cysts were found in the glottal area. The cysts may be located on the vocal fold, or on the wave or edge of the subglottal area. Stroboscopy is a technique which is clinically helpful, especially when a differential diagnostic of vocal fold nodules is required. Whenever there is evidence of a cyst with tissue growth on the corresponding vocal fold, the main clinical symptom is the differing sizes and configurations. Vocal fold cysts are mainly one-sided and mostly located in the superficial layer of the lamina propria (Figure 5.22 a–d).

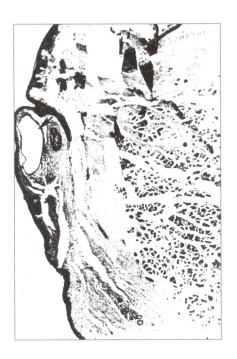

Figure 5.22a
One-sided vocal fold cyst.
Histology (according to Hirano in
Sataloff, 1997); the superficial
layer of the lamina propria and
the epithelium are affected –
probably the deep layer is
reached.

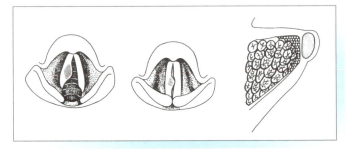

Figure 5.22b
Diagram (according to Hirano
and Bless, 1993); the superficial
layer of the lamina propria
(cover) is affected.

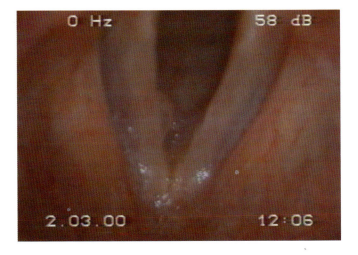

Figure 5.22c
Videolaryngoscopic findings in
respiration position.

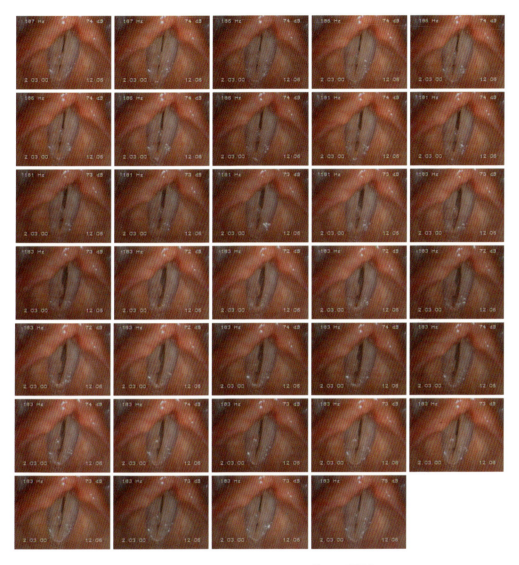

Figure 5.22d

One-sided vocal fold cyst; stroboscopic video sequence:

Glottal closure: along the entire glottis

Amplitude: right normal to reduced, left normal

Symmetry: without marked phase shift

Periodicity: periodic

Regularity: normal vibration pattern

Mucosal wave: right reduced, left normal

Phonatoric immobility: not present

Supraglottic constriction: not present.

The cyst is characterized as a balloon-like form with a liquid-filled sack. A posterior or anterior imcomplete glottal closure may appear; a one- or two-sided hourglass-shaped glottis may also appear. As a result, increased vocal fold stiffness with incomplete glottal closure occurs during phonation. The amplitude is reduced on the affected side and a symmetry during the vibration process can no longer be seen. The mucosal wave is reduced on the affected side. In cases of cysts below the free vocal fold edge, more likely located in the subglottal area, there is a type of cyst shift within the mucosal wave which takes place during phonation. Here the cyst may also be shifted beyond the free edge of the vocal fold on to the surface of the vocal fold independent of the cyst location. During the process of vocal fold vibration, subglottal cysts may move.

5.7.5 Vocal fold polyps

Stroboscopic findings are dependent on the size and location of vocal fold polyps. Assuming that the vocal fold polyp is located in the superficial layer of the lamina propria (Figure 5.23 a–d), there will be various characteristics present which reveal an insufficient glottal closure, a decreased amplitude, and an asymmetry of the mucosal wave on the affected side. Thus no phonatoric immobility will occur. When the polyp is squeezed between the vocal folds during phonation, the stroboscopic movement process may be stopped on both sides. In contrast, when an hourglass-shaped glottis appears, the stroboscopic features of the anterior incomplete glottal closure may differ from findings within the posterior area. After phonosurgical procedures to improve the voice, the vibration mode should normalize within a few days of operative treatment. This indicates that a pre- and post-operative stroboscopic assessment in the case of removal of vocal fold polyps should be undertaken.

5.7.6 Reinke's oedema

The causes of Reinke's oedema remain unclear. Predisposed factors cited are smoking and heavy voice use. Females are more affected than males. Reinke's oedema tends to appear during middle or old age. Pathological changes are found in the superficial layer of the lamina propria: the Reinke's space. Through oedematous deposit, stiffness of the cover is reduced and mass is increased. This leads to an increase of vibrating mucosa, whereby the vibration process of both vocal folds may be affected. An increase in mass and effects on the vibration movement are causes of decreased fundamental frequency of the voice and hoarseness. During phonation a complete

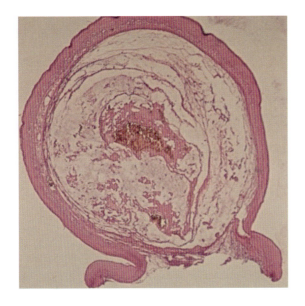

Figure 5.23a
One-sided vocal fold polyp. Histology; oedematous-gelatinous and vascularized thickening of the stroma covered with epithelium (after Kleinsasser, CD-ROM).

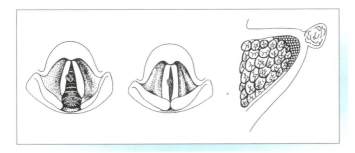

Figure 5.23b
Diagrammatic representation of Figure 5.23a; the superficial layer of the lamina propria (cover) is affected (after Hirano and Bless, 1993).

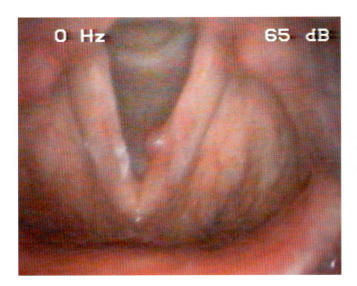

Figure 5.23c
Videolaryngoscopic findings in respiration position.

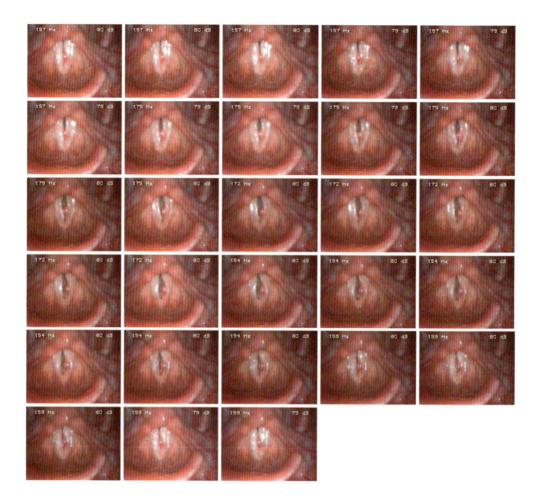

Figure 5.23d

One-sided vocal fold polyp;
stroboscopic video sequence:

Glottal closure: posterior gap

Amplitude: right normal, left
  increased

Symmetry: asymmetric with marked
  phase shift

Periodicity: periodic

Regularity: normal vibration pattern,
  light longitudinal waveform of the
  right vocal fold

Mucosal wave: left reduced to absent

phonatoric immobility: not present

Supraglottic constriction: not present.

glottal closure normally occurs, with partially aperiodic, asymmetric and often irregular vibrations. The mucosal wave appears especially prominent and is occasionally vertically moving, even if the vibration amplitude is reduced along the horizontal plane. A phonatoric immobility is not observed in the case of a Reinke's oedema (Figure 5.24 a–d).

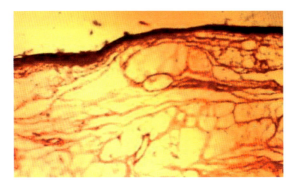

Figure 5.24a
Reinke's oedema. Histology. Oedema of the subepithelium. Epithelium flat (after Behrendt: histological archive of the ENT-University hospital, Leipzig).

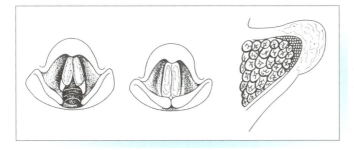

Figure 5.24b
Diagram. The superficial layer of the lamina propria (cover) is concerned (Hirano and Bless 1993).

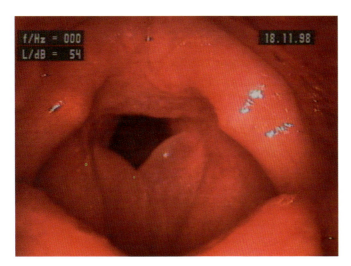

Figure 5.24c
Videolaryngoscopic findings in respiration position.

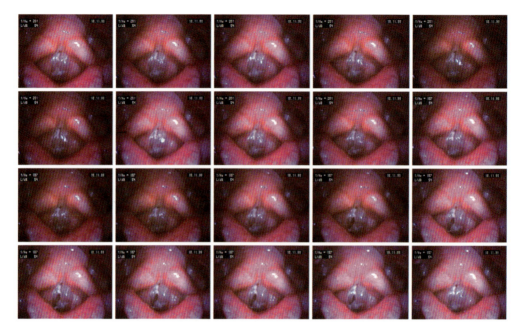

Figure 5.24d

Reinke's oedema; stroboscopic video sequence:

Glottal closure: complete

Amplitude: reduced

Symmetry: not determined

Periodicity: aperiodic

Regularity: irregular waveform

Mucosal wave: not determined

phonatoric immobility: not present

Supraglottic constriction: anterior-posterior

5.7.7 Sulcus vocalis

Sulcus vocalis can appear on one or both sides. It can affect the entire length of the afflicted vocal fold or be restricted to one section only. The retraction on the medial vocal fold edge includes only the outer (superficial) layer of the lamina propria (Figure 5.25 a–d). By studying the location and the histological picture of the sulcus vocalis, a deduction of stroboscopic features may be made. The glottal closure may occasionally be no longer seen in the case of one or two-sided sulcus glottidis. The amplitude is reduced depending on the dimensions of the sulcus. Symmetry may be seen only in the case of a double-sided sulcus vocalis. Along part of the sulcus, a mucosal wave can no longer be seen. Depending on the prominence and

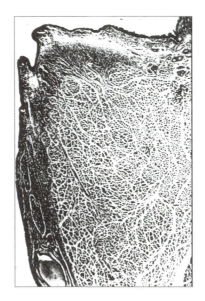

Figure 5.25a
Sulcus vocalis
Histology; the superficial layer is affected; tight, collagenous fibres and rare capillaries are usually present (after Hirano in Sataloff, 1997).

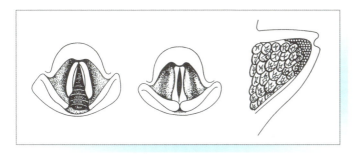

Figure 5.25b
Diagram; the superficial layer of the lamoina propria (cover) is affected (after Hirano and Bless, 1993).

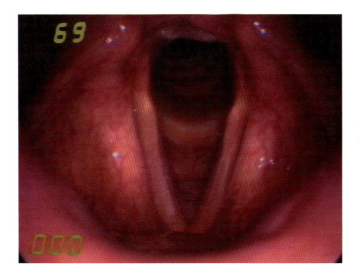

Figure 5.25c
Videolaryngoscopic findings in respiration position.

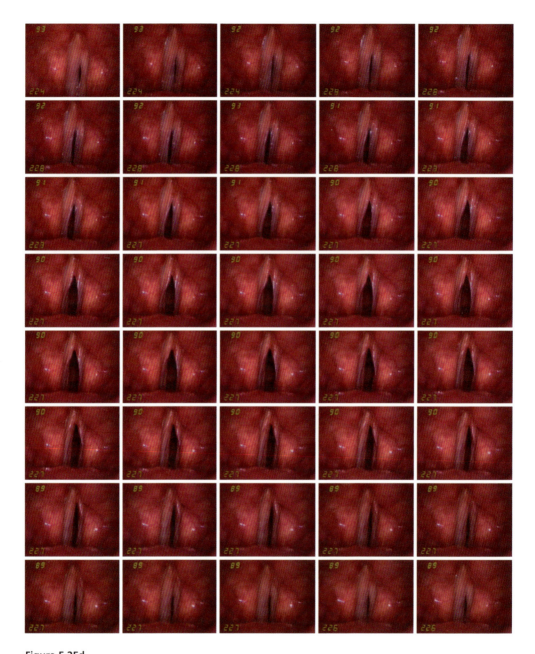

Figure 5.25d

Sulcus vocalis; stroboscopic
video sequence:
Glottal closure: incomplete
  (arch-shaped)
Amplitude: normal
Symmetry: amplitude normal with
  phase shift

Periodicity: periodic
Regularity: normal waveform
Mucosal wave: normal
phonatoric immobility: not present
Supraglottic constriction: not
  present

location, the sulcus vocalis may have very different effects on the voice quality. Pronounced hoarseness is noticeable sometimes, while at other times no influence on the voice may be detected.

5.7.8 Paralysis of the laryngeal nerves

It is not possible to differentiate between paralysis of the vagal and recurrent nerve using laryngostroboscopy. In contrast however, there are stroboscopic features which allow differentiation between a paresis of the N. laryngeus superior and a paresis of the N. laryngeus.

5.7.8.1 N. laryngeus superior

Paresis of the N. laryngeus superior is characterized by dysphonia, limited ability to sing in higher frequencies and rotation of the arytenoid region on the paralysed side during higher phonation. Since the movement between the phonation and respiration position is maintained, other pathological stroboscopic assessment criteria occur, in contrast to paresis of the N. laryngeus recurrens.

According to Dursun et al. (1996), among 126 patients with a paresis and paralysis of the N. laryngeus superior, 84.9% experienced an amplitude asymmetry in the stroboscopic vibratory pattern and only 15.1% experienced a symmetry. Further stroboscopic features may be seen in Table 5.7. An electromyographical assessment is indispensable despite indications of clinical and stroboscopic findings.

Table 5.7 Videostroboscopic findings in the case of a paresis and paralysis of the N. laryngeus superior (n = 126) (Dursun et al., 1996)

Amplitude			Glissando		
asymmetry	107	(84.9%)	normal	36	(28.6%)
symmetry	19	(15.1%)	limited	90	(71.4%)
Phase			**Amplitude**		
asymmetry	92	(73%)	normal	22	(17.3%)
symmetry	34	(27%)	reduced	86	(68.2%)
			increased	18	(14.3%)
Periodicity					
present	51	(40.5%)	**Mucosal wave**		
partly present	66	(52.4%)	normal	27	(21.4%)
not present	9	(7.1%)	shortened	87	(69.1%)
			expanded	12	(9.5%)
Glottal closure					
complete	35	(27.7%)			
incomplete	70	(55.5%)			
posterior triangle	21	(16.7%)			

5.7.8.2 N. laryngeus recurrens

It has been shown that the paralysed vocal fold always reveals a vibration pattern in the phonation level, although the vocal fold stands still in one position. The vibration pattern is always pathological, and stroboscopic symptoms are dependent on the position of the paralysed vocal fold; it can be further categorized as either flaccid or stiff. Due to many influencing factors, this further categorization as flaccid or stiff takes on a critical value (see Table 5.8). Besides a reduced range of rough mobility, the results of a vocal fold paralysis include a limited ability to adjust the muscle tonus to the pitch. In addition, atrophy of the affected muscles normally occurs.

Table 5.8 Configuration of the glottis with peripheral vocal cord paralysis (Boehme, 2000)
The position of paralysed vocal folds depends on
• degree of denervation • degree of reinnervation • contraction of affected muscles • atrophy of affected muscles • compensation of laryngeal movements • type of progress, e.g. acute or chronic • variable anastomosis between N. laryngeus superior, Ramus internus and N. laryngeus recurrens, N. laryngeus superior, Ramus internus and Ramus externus and N. laryngeus superior, Ramus externus and N. laryngeus recurrens

Using stroboscopy, the examiner will search systematically for detailed findings such as failure of glottal closure, amplitude, symmetry, periodicity, regularity, mucosal waves and supraglottal constriction. In the case of vocal fold paresis, a phonatoric immobility does not occur without a simultaneous infiltrative process (Figures 5.26 and 5.27).

Glottal closure

Due to the one- or two-sided vocal fold paralysis, an incomplete glottal closure or a clearly shortened closed phase may be seen in the stroboscopic picture.

Amplitude

In the case of stiff vocal fold paralysis the amplitude is reduced. In the case of flaccid paralysis the amplitude is increased. Thus the amplitude is pathological in comparison with healthy vocal folds. Additionally, the amplitudes are dependent on the position of the paralysed vocal fold (Fex, 1970).

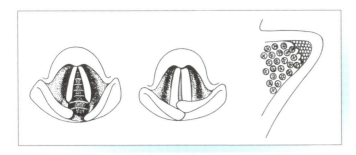

Figure 5.26a
Flaccid paresis of the left
recurrent nerve, condition after
bronchial carcinoma.
Diagram; the muscle (body) is
affected (Hirano and Bless,
1993).

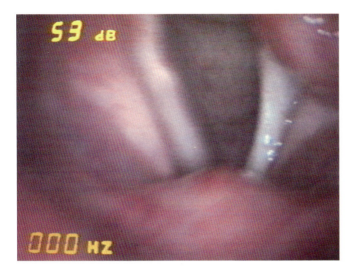

Figure 5.26b
Male, 70 years.
Flaccid paresis of the left
recurrent nerve, condition after
bronchial carcinoma.
Video laryngoscopy during
respiration: right vocal fold with
good rough mobility; left vocal
fold flaccid paresis.

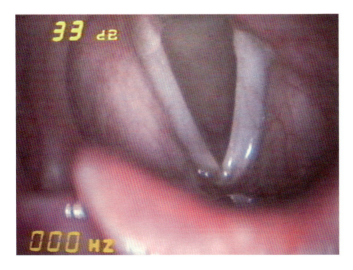

Figure 5.27a
Female, 56 years.
Idiopathic stiff left vocal fold
paralysis. Video laryngoscopy
during respiration.

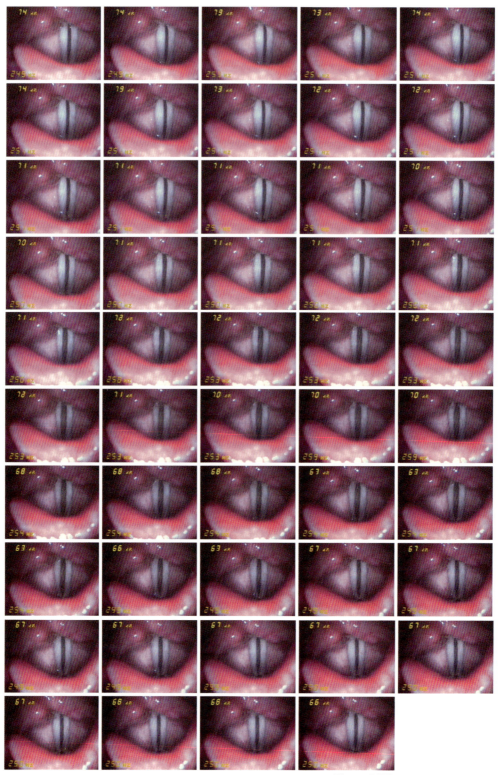

Figure 5.27b

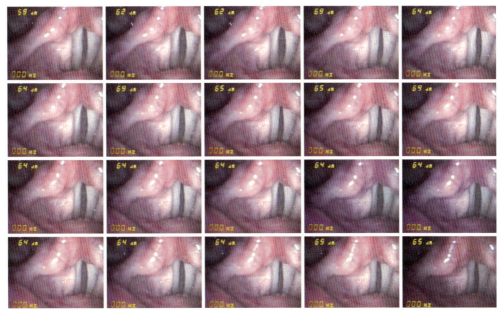

Figure 5.27b (page 80)

Idiopathic stiff vocal fold paralysis
left, female, 56 years
Videostroboscopy (at least two
  periods):
Glottal closure: incomplete
Amplitude: reduced
Symmetry: Reduced on the right
  side, reduced on left side, distinct
  phase shift
Periodicity: periodic (hard to assess)
Regularity: normal wave form
Mucosal wave: reduced
Phonatoric immobility: not present
Supraglottic constriction: anterior-
  posterior.

Figure 5.27c

Videostroboscopy:
Glottal closure: incomplete
Amplitude: left normal, right
  increased
Symmetry: amplitude asymmetrical
  with pronounced phase shift
Periodicity: aperiodic
Regularity: irregular resp.
  unable to assess
Mucosal wave: cannot be assessed
  due to insufficient glottal closure
Phonatoric immobility: not present
Supraglottal constriction: anterior-
  posterior.

Additional comments

Vocal fold vibrations are present only slightly on the right of the non-paretic side. The reason may be found in the insufficient analytic capabilities of the human eye when viewing still images. In contrast, vibrations are more recognizable on video.

Symmetry

In the case of one-sided vocal fold paralysis, asymmetric stroboscopic findings can generally be determined. These may appear not only as asymmetry of amplitude, but also as a phase shift.

Regularity

Seeman (1921) described for the first time that noticeable upwards movements of the paralysed vocal fold, like a flag flapping in the wind, could be determined, especially for flaccid vocal fold paralysis. This flutter movement of the paralysed vocal fold is also described as 'vertical vibration component'.

Mucosal waves

In the case of one-sided vocal fold paralysis, a regular mucosal wave on the same side is seen only when both vocal folds have the same stiffness.

1. Sercarz et al. (1992); Harries and Morrison (1996); Woo (1997) describe a change in mucosal wave speed in contrast to the healthy side in the case of a one-sided vocal fold paralysis. Asymmetry of the mucosal wave with phase shift is the most common finding. The travelling wave motion is faster on a healthy vocal fold, which leads to a difference in phases between the two vocal folds. Additionally, the wave motion on the healthy side reveals a larger mucosal deflection. The tension of the paralysed vocal folds and the phonated frequency (low – high) must be considered.
2. The mucosal wave is apparently not dependent on the presence or absence of innervation. A much more decisive role is played by tension, position and form of the vocal folds, as well as subglottal pressure.

Patients with vocal fold paralysis of course may develop a mucosal wave even after surgical medialization of the vocal fold, even if a denervation with EMG criteria is proven (Kokesh et al., 1993). During such examinations it must be considered that the glottis configuration is dependent on many factors in the case of vocal fold paralysis (Table 5.8).

Phonatoric immobility

Normally a phonatoric immobility is not seen in the case of vocal fold paralysis. In addition to a series of other distinctive features which may appear to be present, the illusion of a one-sided phonatoric immobility may occur during a biphonation (different frequency behaviour on the vocal fold sides). Through a change in pitch it is possible to recognize vocal fold vibration immediately and realize that a true phonatoric immobility has not occurred.

5.7.8.3 Differential diagnosis: arytenoid cartilage luxation

In the case of a one-sided arytenoid cartilage luxation (dislocation), the affected side will experience missing rough motility of the vocal fold, although a paralysis of the N. laryngeus recurrens cannot be proved. Normally there is an especially pronounced shift of the proc. vocalis of the arytenoid cartilage.

The findings may be normal: a normal glottal closure, a symmetry and a regular mucosal wave. A phonatoric immobility is not present. The findings thus vary in principle from those of a one-sided paralysis of the recurrent laryngeal nerve.

In the case of an arytenoid cartilage luxation, however, a pathological vibration pattern with asymmetrical amplitude may be observed with stroboscopic imagery; reasons are the varying muscle tone of the M. vocalis and M. thyroarytaenoideus.

In terms of differential diagnostics, however, the electromyographical findings are decisive (Table 5.9).

Table 5.9 Arytenoid cartilage luxation – one-sided vocal fold paralysis: differential diagnosis

Rigid endoscopy	Arytenoid cartilage luxation	Vocal fold paralysis
	No mobility of vocal fold, arytenoid cartilage: (not only Wrisberg-Santorini cartilage) very noticeably dislocated	No mobility of vocal fold, arytenoid cartilage not dislocated (but possibly Wrisberg-Santorini cartilage)
Stroboscopy	Normal and/orpathologic	Pathologic
Electromyography	Normal	Pathologic
Computer tomogram	Arytenoid cartilage: very noticeably dislocated	Subglottal space flattened on the paretic side

5.7.9 Hyperkeratosis, leukoplakia

Hyperkeratosis

Lesions may appear on one or both sides or appear exophytically within the vocal fold area. Hyperkeratosis stems from the epithelium and includes the superficial layer of the lamina propria. In cases of flat hyperkeratosis, the stroboscopic vibration abilities of vocal folds are not limited. Due to the stiffness and increase in mass within the vocal fold, an incomplete and irregular glottal closure may be observed stroboscopically in the case of extended hyperkeratosis. Here amplitudes are reduced on one or both sides (depending on the location of the hyperkeratosis); additionally an asymmetry may be observed. Also, a mucosal wave is not present on the affected side (Hirano and Bless, 1993). Also in the case of extended hyperkeratosis, a phonatoric immobility is purely mechanical (without invasive infiltration). In unclear cases an excisional biopsy is usually necessary.

Leukoplakia

Leukoplakia is a description given to a white patch in the vocal fold mucosa. This can be due to various conditions including hyperkeratosis, hyperplasia, dysplasia and carcinoma in situ. The sections shown as white in the vocal fold mucosa, Figure 5.28 a–d, may evolve as a pre-malignant form into a squamous epithilium carcinoma through chemical toxins (especially tobacco and alcohol consumption). These epithelial hyperplasias lead to a dysphonic voice if located in the glottal area. Since normally in the case of leukoplakia there is no invasive growth, there is also normally no evidence of a phonatoric immobility. If this does occur, an infiltrative process – such as a carcinoma in situ or a vocal fold carcinoma – may follow (see section 5.7.10).

For simple squamous epithelial hyperplasia (Level 1) at the pre-operative stage (prior to excisive biopsy), vocal fold vibration is not, or is only slightly, limited in stroboscopic terms. The thicker the epithelium, the stiffer it is and the more vibratory ability is limited; here the mucosal wave practically disappears (Arndt 1994).

5.7.10 Carcinoma in situ, vocal fold carcinoma

The most important early symptom of vocal fold carcinoma is hoarseness. The most common symptom of other organic and functional laryngeal disorders is also dysphonia. From a therapeutic voice

Practical fact

Stroboscopy provides a great deal of information for diagnostics, differential diagnostics and observation of the progress of vocal fold carcinoma.

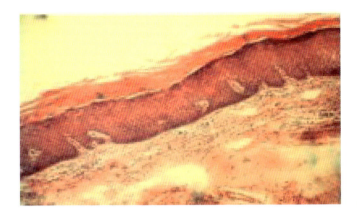

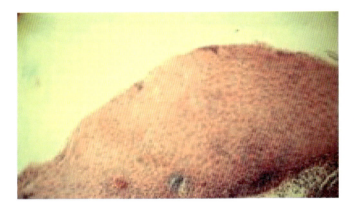

Figure 5.28a
One-sided epithelial hyperplasia/dysplasia (leukoplakia).

Histology
top: hyper- and parakeratotic epithelium (clinically leukoplakia)

middle: considerable keratosis of the epithelium

bottom: peg-form growth into deeper regions; light to moderate dysplasia (after Behrendt: histological archive of the ENT-University hospital, Leipzig).

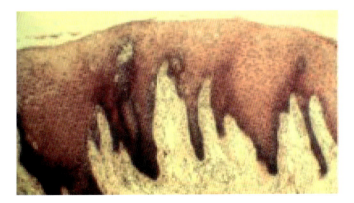

Figure 5.28b

Diagrammatic representation of Figure 5.28a

epithelium → superficial layer of the lamina propria (cover) is affected (after Hirano and Bless 1993).

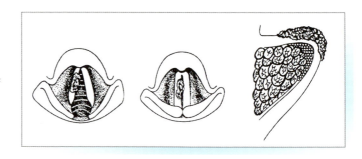

Figure 5.28c

Video laryngoscopy in respiration position.

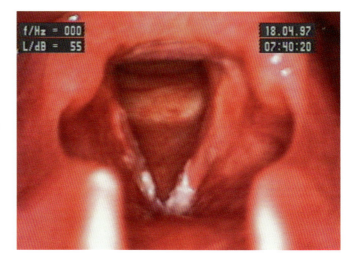

perspective in particular, it is thus extremely important to differentiate malignant laryngeal tumours from other voice disorders, in particular with the aid of laryngostroboscopy. The main laryngological focus is the use of stroboscopy in cases of chronic hyperplastic laryngitis, hyperkeratosis, leukoplakia, malignant laryngeal disease (carcinoma in situ, vocal fold carcinoma) as well as the care of these disorders.

Laryngeal stroboscopy allows detection of early stages of infiltrative alterations in the glottal area. These early stages may be missed in the macromorphological evidence of image-producing techniques such as computer tomography (CT) and magnetic resonance imaging (MRI) (Bigenzahn et al., 1998).

As a feature of an infiltrative vocal fold process, the decreased amplitude and mucosal waves may be characterized as a phonatoric immobility.

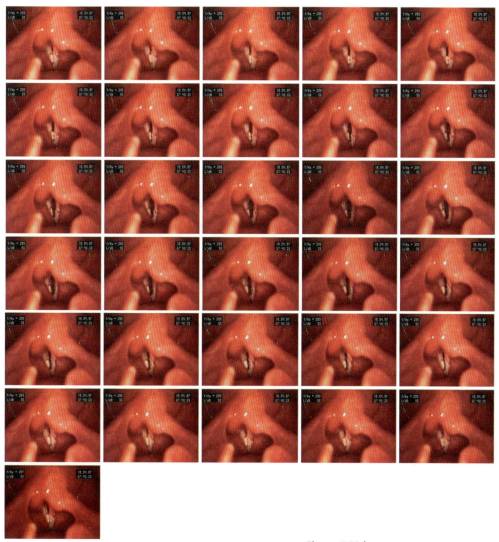

Figure 5.28d
Epithelial hyperplasia/dysplasia
(leukoplakia); stroboscopic video
sequence:
Glottal closure: incomplete, posterior gap
Amplitude: reduced to normal
Symmetry: present
Periodicity: periodic
Regularity: normal waveform
Mucosal wave: reduced in the anterior
 third on both sides
Phonatoric immobility: not present
Supraglottic constriction: anterior-
posterior.

In an extended sense, Bigenzahn et al. (1998) can provide the following stroboscopic evidence of an infiltrative vocal fold process:

- reduction of vocal fold amplitude
- decrease of mucosal wave
- phonatoric immobility; amplitudes and mucosal waves are absent. The reduced range of motor activity of vocal folds is possible when changing between the adduction and abduction positions.

Carcinoma in situ (pre-invasive carcinoma)

Stroboscopic experience with histological evidence reveals that this is an early stage which is detectable outside of macromorphological evidence using CT and MRI; this is very rarely mentioned in literature available worldwide. In 1998 Bigenzahn et al. described two cases involving carcinoma in situ:

Case 1

Using rigid endoscopy for high-grade leukoplakia on both vocal folds there was a clearly reduced mucosal wave and a reduction of amplitudes.

Case 2

Using rigid endoscopy there was a visible thickening of the right vocal fold. Now a phonatoric immobility may be shown by stroboscopic means. With the help of computed tomography with an axial view with I.V. means of contrast medium, a regular, even-sided presentation of vocal folds was achieved without a tumour for the right vocal fold or the need for pathological contrast stain.

Vocal fold carcinoma

Epithelial hyperplasia of the vocal folds more rarely reaches deeper structures. As soon as a carcinoma invades the basal membrane (see Chapter 1, section 1.1) it is no longer a carcinoma in situ, by definition. If the morphological structural alterations include more than three-quarters of the membraneous vocal fold, a complete phonatoric immobility of vocal folds occurs in the stroboscopic image, that is, amplitudes and mucosal waves are no longer present (Zhao et al.,

Practical fact

According to these two case reports varying stroboscopic results may be expected in the case of carcinoma in situ.

1991). In contrast, it is well known that phonatoric immobility always occurs in the stroboscopic image during the early stages of vocal fold carcinoma due to deep infiltration via ligament in the M. vocalis (Colden et al., 2001); Hirano and Bless, 1993; Sessions et al., 1992) (Figure 5.30 a–c).

Excision biopsy and stroboscopy

As indispensable as an excision biopsy may be in solidifying the diagnosis of 'vocal fold carcinoma', the test may yet be unsuitable in some cases where dysphonia is unclear. The excision biopsy may considerably delay the healing process of the dysphonia, should there be an infection instead of a carcinoma. The stroboscopic vibration pattern of vocal folds are also naturally affected by a excision biopsy.

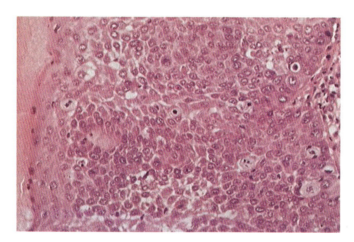

Figure 5.29a
Carcinoma in situ, left. Histology; broadened epithelium; mitoses reach the superficial epthelial layer without symptoms of invasion (after Lehmann et al., 1981).

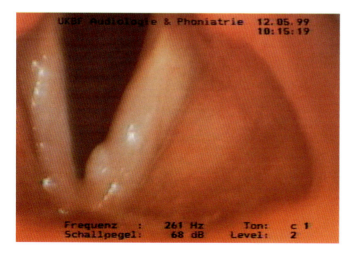

Figure 5.29b
Videolaryngoscopy in respiration position.

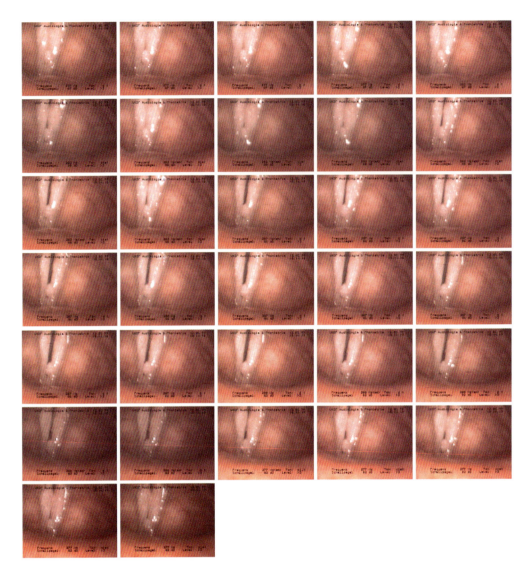

Figure 5.29c
Carcinoma in situ, left
Stroboscopic video sequence:
Glottis closure: complete
Amplitude: reduced
Symmetry: present with slight phase shift
Periodicity: periodic
Regularity: normal waveform
Mucosal wave: reduced in the anterior
  third on both sides
Phonatoric immobility: not present
Supraglottic constriction: not present.

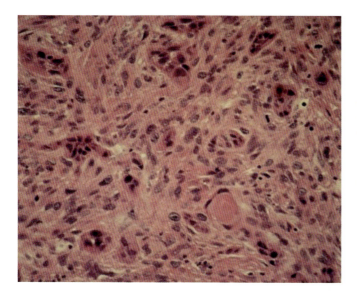

Figure 5.30a
Vocal fold carcinoma right. Histology; moderately differentiated epidermoid carcinoma; atypical cells with two nodular foci (after Lehmann et al., 1981) .

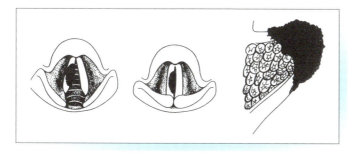

Figure 5.30b
Diagrammatic representation of figure 5.30a. Epithelium → lamina propria → muscle (cover) are affected (after Hirano and Bless 1993).

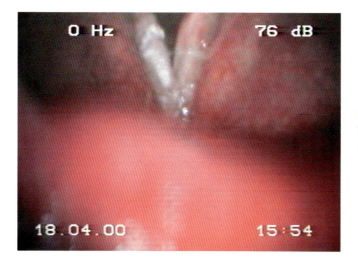

Figure 5.30c
Videolaryngoscopic findings in respiration position.

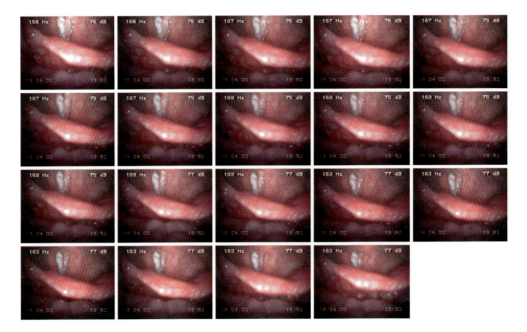

Figure 5.30d

Vocal fold carcinoma right: Stroboscopic video sequence:

Glottis closure: incomplete (posterior gap)

Amplitude: right side markedly reduced, left side reduced

Symmetry: not present

Periodicity: periodic

Regularity: right waveform not determined, left normal

Mucosal wave: right not present, left reduced

Phonatoric immobility: right complete, left not present

Supraglottic constriction: anterior-posterior.

Thus a stroboscopic assessment should be made prior to a excision biopsy with glottal findings where there is a suspicion of T_1 or T_2.

Stroboscopic examination with radiation therapy

During radiation therapy, stroboscopy allows examination of the healing process and allows elimination of local relapse. For this reason it is necessary to perform regular stroboscopic examination after completion of radio-oncological treatment.

The recurrence of vibration amplitudes and mucosal waves in the case of advanced phonatoric immobility after primary radiation therapy for in situ carcinoma or T_1 to T_2 is a good prognostic sign.

> **Practical fact**
>
> Stroboscopy plays a supportive role in monitoring patients receiving radiation treatment. A relapse is present if a phonatoric immobility occurs again after initial return of vibration amplitudes and mucosal waves.

Karduck and Bartholome (1976) observed 45 patients with glottal carcinoma (T_1, T_1a and tumour in situ) after radium contact radiation. At three weeks at the earliest, and nine months at the latest, a normal phonatoric vocal fold vibration was seen during stroboscopic examination. Tsunoda et al. (1997) also determined a reoccurrence of mucosal waves in 10 patients with T_1 tumours one year after radiation therapy. In contrast, Sopko (1980), Lehmann et al. (1988) and Dworkin et al. (1999) described limited or absence of mucosal waves, irregularities, insufficient glottal closure and amplitude reduction due to scarring and fibrous degeneration and after radiation therapy.

If there is phonatoric immobility after primary radiation therapy, this does not prove a residual or relapse tumour according to Wallesch et al. (1991). In addition to relapses, there may be infection-prone or a scarred residue after an excision biopsy.

Differential diagnosis

A case of acute and chronic *laryngitis* may lead to a phonatoric immobility for a limited time (approx. 8–14 days). During longer phonatoric immobility, a *vocal fold tuberculosis* mainly occurring on one side should always be considered in addition to glottis carcinoma (see also section 5.7.11). During the post-operative period after *vocal fold nodule*, *polyp* or *papilloma removal* a phonatoric vocal fold immobility may be seen for weeks or months. Also in the case of a negligible reduction of vibration ability, a superficial process such as a carcinoma in situ (see above) may not be entirely excluded. Due to possible partial immobility, rigid videoendoscopic examination and stroboscopic progress monitoring within the entire pitch range are recommended for early diagnosis (Wendler et al., 1996).

5.7.11 Vocal fold tuberculosis

The leading clinical symptoms of laryngeal tuberculosis are dysphonia and/or odynophagy. Using stroboscopy, phonatoric immobility may be observed. Differentiation of phonatoric immobility in the case of glottal carcinoma is not possible. Thus an excision biopsy is necessary in the case of phonatoric immobility. The simultaneous occurrence of laryngeal tuberculosis and laryngeal carcinoma must be taken into consideration.

Various stroboscopic findings have been described for laryngeal tuberculosis. Agarwal and Bais (1998) mention vibratory asymmetry, reduction of amplitude, and additional reduction of mucosal waves. Since the leading symptom of vocal fold tuberculosis is phonatoric immobility with lack of amplitude and mucosal waves, glottal carcinoma must always be considered. In this case, stroboscopic findings may support the indications of a test excision. In contrast, stroboscopic findings alone without further pneumological diagnosis are insufficient (Pease et al., 1997). Stroboscopic findings may be applied after glottal carcinoma is excluded for the purposes of monitoring progress of vocal fold tuberculosis.

5.7.12 Central voice disorders

Our knowledge of stroboscopic findings in cases of central voice disorders is not yet complete. Experience has been gathered especially in relation to assessments of dysarthria. Reference is made to the observations of Schröter-Morasch (1998). In stroboscopic terms, the following criteria are critical:

- reduced glottal closure
- increased opening quotient
- reduced opening quotient
- irregularity (right/left)
- expanded amplitudes (right/left)
- reduced amplitudes (right/left)
- reduced mucosal wave (right/left)
- limited pitch variation
- limited loudness variation.

Two diagnoses involving central voice disorders are now described: a common and a rare diagnosis.

Parkinson's disease
Prevalence is 100–200 per 100,000 people.
Stelzig et al. (1999) found the following stroboscopic characteristics for Parkinson's disease (Figure 5.31):

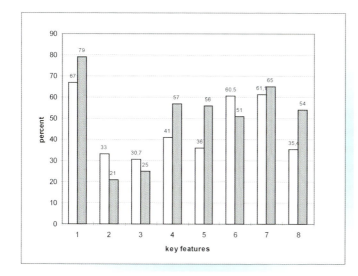

Figure 5.31
Key features of alterations in laryngeal findings for female patients (light bars) and male patients (dark bars) with Parkinson's disease (according to Stelzig et al., 1999).
1 = symmetric abduction and adduction of vocal folds
2 = asymmetrical abduction and adduction of vocal folds
3 = laryngeal tremor
4 = false vocal fold hypertrophy on both sides
5 = vocalis atrophy on both sides
6 = insufficient glottal closure
7 = pathologically changed vibration amplitudes
8 = pathologically changed mucosal waves

Spasmodic dysphonia
This is a rare disorder with an occurrence of about 3.5 per 1 million people. Stroboscopic characteristics for adductor-type dysphonia are variable and may only support the diagnosis of a spasmodic dysphonia. Thus the glottal closure is not disturbed. Amplitude and symmetry may also be normal. Yet the findings varied between an extreme hyperfunctional phonation with an extended closed phase and supraglottal constriction on one hand, and normal phonation on the other hand.

5.8 Functional voice disorders

Functional dysphonia is a voice disorder characterized by voice sound disturbance and limitation of voice output, without evidence of

Practical fact

Stroboscopic findings for adductor-type spasmodic dysphonia only occasionally lead to the target diagnosis.

pathological primary organic alterations of anatomical structures involved in voice production. Functional variations may appear in the sense of 'too much' (hyperfunctional dysphonia) or 'too little' (hypofunctional dysphonia). Primarily affected are subglottal pressure (breathing apparatus activity) and glottal resistance (mass or mass distribution and tension or vocal fold stiffness); the muscular position of the vocal tract and even the entire body may be affected. According to Fröschels, functional vocal disorders may originate in different regions (Figure 5.32). Stroboscopic images reveal functional laryngeal disorders. This means that not every voice disorder can be identified as a result of noticeable stroboscopic findings.

Figure 5.32

Localization of hyperfunctional symptoms in the respiratory, phonatory and articulatory system (Fröschels, 1937, modified by Boehme, 2003).

Key

1	Subglottis
2	Glottis
3 + 4	Pharynx
5	Soft palate
6	Tongue
7	Lips
8	Jaw

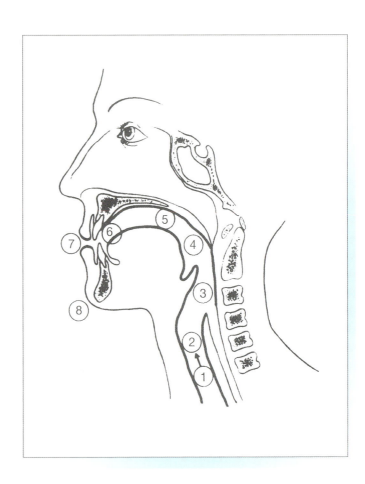

5.8.1 Hyperfunctional dysphonia

Hyperfunctional dysphonia is by far the most common functional voice disorder, and affects mainly males. Symptoms such as external appearance with hyperlordosis, a strong handshake and high thoracic breathing pattern belong to the hyperfunctional dysphonia condition. Additionally, there normally occurs an increased fundamental frequency of the voice, a pathologically hard voice onset and a middle-grade increase in voice capability with a tendency towards increased voice loudness. According to Fröschels (1937), hyperfunctional dysphonia may be localized on various anatomical structures. Accordingly, Fröschels identifies ten types of hyperfunctional dysphonia and Boehme (1997) identifies 12 various forms. Only those types of hyperfunctional dysphonia with subglottal, glottal and direct supraglottal localization affect stroboscopic imagery. In the case of velar and lingual hyperfunctionality, the articulation reaction on the larynx is often changed so much through the examination method (extension of tongue during rigid endoscopy or laryngeal mirror), that a spontaneous improvement of the voice sound and normal glottal vibration pattern occurs. If these patients are examined transnasally using fibre-endoscopic methods, then a typical appearance of hyperfunctional dysphonia may also be recognized using stroboscopic methods. With laryngeal localization, there is laryngoscopic evidence of muscle activity in the form of hypopharyngeal constriction, an anterior-posterior constriction of the supraglottis, a protrusion of the petiolus, as well as false vocal folds. During stroboscopic examination of hyperfunctional dysphonia, an extended closed phase is usually seen even when voice intensity is small (Figure 5.33). Vibration amplitudes appear reduced in contrast to normal voices.

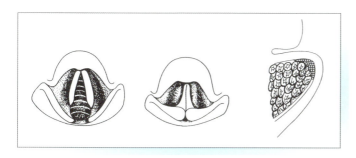

Figure 5.33a
Diagrammatic representation of Hyperfunctional dysphonia; no organic pathology (Hirano and Bless, 1993).

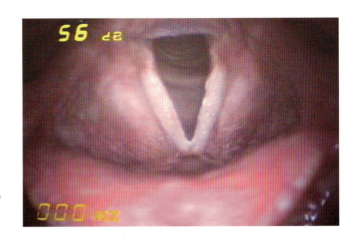

Figure 5.33b
Videolaryngoscopic findings in respiration position.

Figure 5.33c (below)
Stroboscopic video sequence; the very long closed phase is typical.

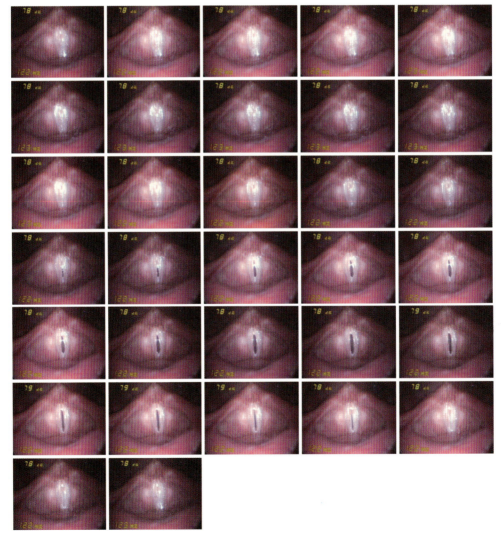

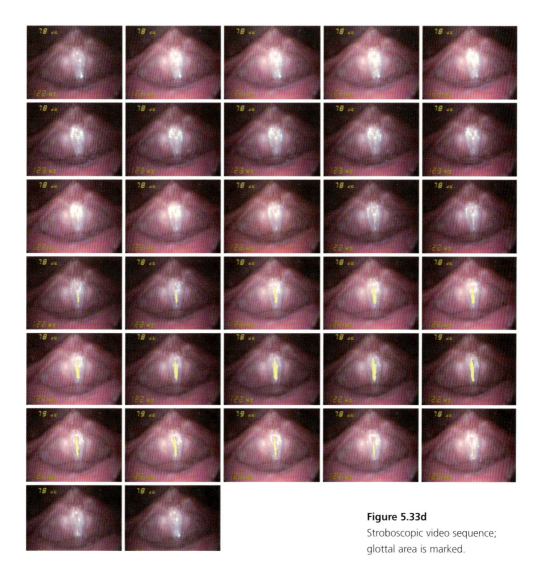

Figure 5.33d
Stroboscopic video sequence;
glottal area is marked.

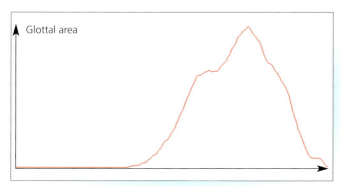

Figure 5.33e
Diagram of the glottal area
during a vibration period, from
Figure 5.33(d); although the
sound is low the closed phase is
very long (glottal area = 0 pixel).

5.8.1.1 False vocal folds

Both the intended false vocal fold voice (e.g. the condition after cordectomy) and the unintended false vocal fold voice as an extreme variation of hyperfunctional dysphony are characterized by voice production on the false vocal folds. This means that the false vocal folds are made to vibrate, and typically a movement process may also be seen on the false vocal folds – as normally seen only on vocal folds. Characteristically the voice sounds considerably rougher, indicating an irregularity of the vibration pattern. Therefore, during stroboscopy it can be expected that the assessment of false vocal fold vibration is limited.

5.8.2 Hypofunctional dysphonia

In contrast to hyperfunctional dysphonia, hypofunctional dysphonia is characterized by a too-low level of activity of the inner and outer laryngeal muscles during phonation. There are no organic alterations to the vocal folds. Vocal fold vibrations feature a glottal closure which is too short or completely lacking. Correspondingly, despite normal loudness, the closed phase is clearly shorter than with a normal voice, and may be reduced to a minimum. In extreme cases this means that the closed phase is limited to the turning point between the closing and opening phase (Figure 5.34). Vocal fold stiffness is reduced overall. For normal subglottal pressure, vibration amplitudes are normal to increased; for reduced subglottal pressure the amplitudes are normal to reduced.

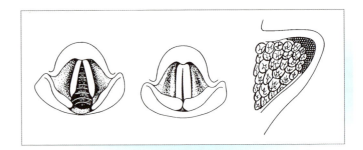

Figure 5.34a

Hypofunctional dysphonia; no organic pathology (Hirano and Bless, 1993).

5.9   Stroboscopy and phonosurgery

Laryngostroboscopy is considered essential in basic examination procedures for phonosurgery. This applies primarily to surgery on vocal folds. In the case of phonosurgical measures, stroboscopic findings must supplemented by a battery of individual tests. These include auditory

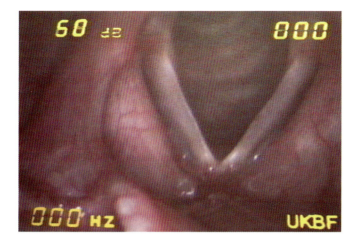

Figure 5.34b
Videolaryngoscopic findings in respiration.

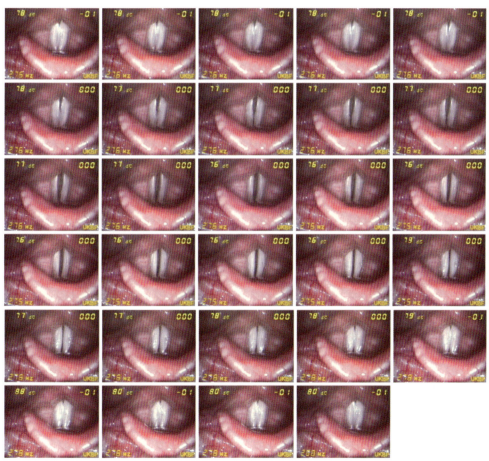

Figure 5.34c
Stroboscopic video sequence; the very short closed phase is typical.

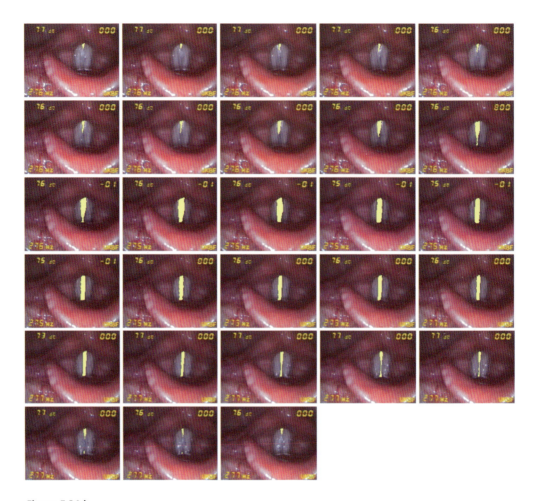

Figure 5.34d
Stroboscopic video sequence;
glottal area is marked.

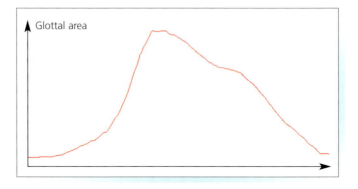

Figure 5.34e
Diagram of glottal area, from
Figure 5.34d, during a vibration
period; the short closed phase is
noticeable (glottal area > 0 pixel).

methods with categorical systems, voice range profile, determination of maximal phonation time and objective voice analyses; if required, aerodynamic techniques and electromyography may also be applied. Tape recordings of the speaking and singing voice completes the examination procedure. Each individual test battery is always required at the pre- and post-operative stage. Basic knowledge of the use of stroboscopic measures to improve the voice have been presented in several individual reports and monographs on phonosurgery (e.g. Ford and Bless, 1991; Gould, Sataloff and Spiegel, 1993; Cornut and Bouchayer, 1999a).

For typical voice disorders, there are various descriptions of pre- and post-operative stroboscopic findings related to voice-improving procedures.

Practical fact

Pre- and post-operative stroboscopic assessment is an essential part of phonosurgery.

Pre- and post-operative test battery according to Zeitels et al., 1997

During visual pre-operative assessment (videolaryngoscopy and video-stroboscopy), a subjective determination of voice quality, an electro-acoustic assessment, and aerodynamic tests may be used. The stroboscopic task is to locate the Reinke's oedema precisely. Given a mucosal wave, the balloon-shaped, enlarged superficial lamina propria may be evaluated. Post-operative stroboscopic analysis should determine the degree to which a normal mucosal wave may be reached with normal amplitudes and phase symmetry.

Pre- and post-operative check according to Murry et al., 1999

They recommend the following stroboscopic assessment criteria for laser surgery treatment of Reinke's oedema:

* the pattern of glottal closure
* symmetry, and
* mucosal waves.

After one post-operative month a mucosal wave was present in all patients (n = 8).

In addition, an acoustic analysis followed with the aid of the Multidimensional Voice Profile (MDVP) analysis program.

Benign tumours and tumour-like alterations of the vocal folds

As in the case of every type of voice-improving measure, microsurgical treatment of vocal fold nodules, cysts, polyps, etc. also requires a pre- and post-operative stroboscopic assessment.

Reinke's oedema

Pre- and post-operative stroboscopic assessment of Reinke's oedema is an important part of phonosurgery. In pre-operative cases it is necessary to make differentiated local findings; in post-operative cases it is necessary to undertake stroboscopic examinations for monitoring the healing process. The goal is to recognize and treat infections in deep layers as early as possible. Permanent post-operative dysphonia may sometimes be traced to a phonatoric immobility, whereby a wound healing disorder, scarring, or an artificial lesion, e.g. through overly-extended tissue or thermic vocal fold damage, may be the cause.

Microflap surgery

Courey et al. (1997) describe medial microflap surgery for benign alterations in vocal folds. Post-operative videostroboscopic assessment revealed that a mucosal wave was present in 16 of 22 patients.

Vocal fold paralysis (paresis of the recurrent nerve)

Videostroboscopic assessments are also indispensable in the pre- and post-operative analysis of microsurgical injection treatment of vocal fold paresis. Various biomaterials are recommended: teflon, preparations containing collagen, hyaluronic acid and fat.

Injection of autologous collagen

Remacle et al. (1999) describe the pre- and post-operative video-stroboscopic findings for treatment of an incomplete glottal closure with one-sided vocal fold paralysis (n = 13), vocal fold atrophy (n = 3), vocal fold scarring (n = 3) and a combination of atrophy (Sulcus vergeture) and scarring (n = 1). Among 13 patients with a vocal fold paralysis, there was stroboscopic evidence of post-operative voice improvement in eight cases.

Indirect vocal fold surgery

Indirect vocal fold surgery methods with local anaesthetic and simultaneous use of stroboscopy requires knowledge of this special technique (e.g. Gross, 1993; Seidner and Wendler, 2000; Wendler, 1983, Wendler et al., 1996).

The advantages of indirect methods may be seen in a three-phase application of stroboscopic assessment methods. In addition to the usual pre-and post-operative stroboscopic analysis, stroboscopic techniques may be applied in an *intraoperative* manner. An advantage is that during an indirect operation a normal vocal fold muscle tone exists. Thus it is possible to perform an intraoperative stroboscopic check of the voice results as well as a vibration analysis.

Thyroplasty

McLean-Muse et al. (2000) performed a stroboscopic assessment of 43 patients who received a thyroplasty, according to Montgomery. In a large percentage of patients normalized stroboscopic findings occurred (see Table 5.10).

Table 5.10 Stroboscopic findings after thyroplasty (McLean-Muse, 2000)		
	Pre-operative	Post-operative
Glottal closure abnormal	37	9
Amplitude abnormal	15	11
Mucosal wave abnormal	16	9

5.10 Sources of error

Stroboscopy may produce false results from a technical, acoustic or clinical point of view. Possible factors of influence may vary widely and they must be taken into consideration at all times.

Perspective errors in rigid endoscopy (Fleischer, Hess and Ludwigs, 1995)

Chapter 3 described the errors in perspective which may be associated with rigid endoscopy. Normally these are not more than 6%. If the patient's head is tilted strongly backwards or forwards, there is a risk that the rigid endoscope is no longer perpendicular to the patient's glottis. In this case errors in perspective may occur.

If the series of flashes is triggered by the microphone signal, the following errors may possibly occur:

* maximum phonation time too short
* voice very hoarse
* biphonation (vibration frequency different for either side).

In order to exclude errors caused by background noise during examination, Fröhlich et al., 1999 recommend using a microphone with a club-shaped recording characteristic.

Assessment of stroboscopic findings in singers without voice disorders

Among 65 professional singers (36 women and 29 men) at the Academy of Vocal Arts (AVA), in Philadelphia, between the ages of 22 and 35, 38 pathological videolaryngostroboscopic findings were made (Elias et al., 1997). The following disorders were discovered:

* 27 × 'reflux laryngitis'
* 2 × vocal fold nodules
* 2 × cysts
* 2 × varicosity
* 4 × asymmetry
* 1 × weakness.

Since subjectively no voice discomfort occurred in professional singers, these findings apparently did not have any significant effect on their professional activities.

Practical fact

Laryngologists and phoniatrists must be aware of the risk of a videostroboscopic misinterpretation for 'healthy-voiced' singers. Despite pathological stroboscopic findings, voice quality may remain unaffected.

6. Electroglottography (EGG)

6.1 Preliminary remarks

Glottography (laryngography) is a non-invasive technique for recording the time cycle of glottal opening and closing movements of the vocal folds during phonation. There are several technical options available for this, whereby primarily *electroglottography (EGG)* (in the UK the term laryngography or electrolaryngography is commonly used) has gained importance as a supplementary technique for other examination methods. *Photoglottography (PGG)* is used together with electroglottography by some medical centres. PGG measures the light permeability of the glottis. The technique formerly described as *ultrasoundglottography* has been further developed as a clinically oriented method and will be described later in Chapter 7 under *sonography* (ultrasound).

6.2 Methodology

In 1957 the biophysicist Fabre developed an impedance method for laryngeal analysis and termed it electroglottography; the test results were named a 'glottogram' (Figures 6.1 and 6.2).

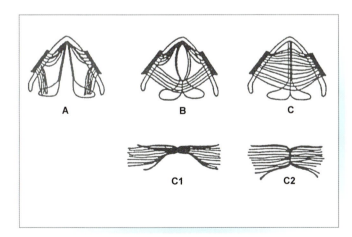

Figure 6.1
Current flow between EGG electrodes at the level of the thyroid cartilage: A = respiration position, B = during open phase of the phonatory cycle, C = during closed phase of the phonatory cycle, C1 and C2 = with different degrees of vocal fold contact during the closed phase (coronal section) (Baken and Orlikoff, 2000).

Stroboscopy and Other Techniques

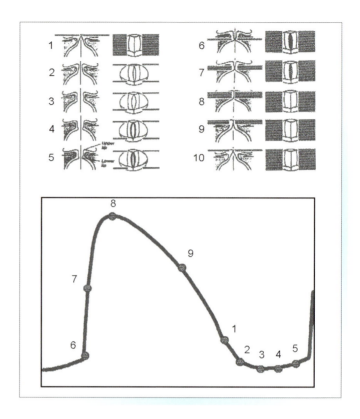

Figure 6.2
Stroboscopy and glottography in compared.
Top left: Progress of one vibration period in coronal section (according to Hirano)
Top right: View from above of the glottis. Grey bars represent the vertical and horizontal conduction path at the vocal fold level.
Bottom: Typical curve progress of an EGG for a healthy-voiced female at habitual fundamental frequency and loudness, modified according to Orlikoff et al. (1999). Waveform upwards: Closing phase = increasing contact. 6 = Beginning of the closing movement; 8 = maximum contact

The examiner should place a plate electrode each on the right and left side of the untreated skin of the neck at the thyroid cartilage level or glottis level. The high-frequency alternating current flowing through the electrodes serves as a carrier frequency for the electro-glottography. The larynx serves as a capacitative resistance which is increased by the opening of the glottis. When the vocal folds draw closer the resistance is reduced. The vocal fold vibration leads to an amplitude modulation of the carrier frequency, which is displayed in the form of an electroglottogram. Unfiltered EGG signals are described as Gx and high-pass filtered signals as Lx. During filtering,

Practical fact

Electroglottography (EGG) allows analysis of vocal fold vibrations in a transcutaneous manner without inspecting the vocal folds. In this way there is no impediment to phonation or articulation. This is the basic difference compared to laryngostroboscopy.

slow impedance changes are eliminated, e.g. head or laryngeal movements. Regardless of whether the vocal folds are in contact, the electroglottogram's highest deflection is the point of time when both vocal folds are closest to each other.

Evaluation

The electroglottogram correlates with the glottal area. In contrast to the optical methods of vibration analysis, the EGG does not allow assessment of the vibration capability of individual vocal folds. Thus EGG is not suitable for early diagnosis of infiltrative processes on the vocal folds. The advantage of the EGG is the possibility of examining glottal vibration patterns without irritation, e.g. from gag reflex. Computer-supported programs are also recommended (e.g. Baken, 1992; Orlikoff, 1998). Hacki (1996) defined the quasi open quotients as having values similar to the open quotients of optical techniques used for vocal fold vibration analysis. He described typical findings for a normal glottal function and both hypofunctional and hyperfunctional dysphonia (Table 6.1).

Table 6.1 Quasi-open quotients (QOQ): average values for people with healthy voices and for patients with functional dysphonia (Hacki, 1989a, 1989b)

	Soft phonation	Loud phonation

Healthy voices
    female
    male
	0.61
	0.65
		0.49
		0.47

Hyperfunction on glottal level	0.54	0.46
Hypofunction on glottal level	0.54	0.61

Typical findings for the laryngeal hyper- and hypofunction are shown in Figures 6.5 and 6.6 (upward waveform: opening movement = reduction of the contact area).

6.3   Application options

The application of dynamic electroglottography (EGG) has a wide variety of uses:

- determination of fundamental frequency
- recognition of periodicity
- assessment of voice register
- determination of speed of vocal fold closing (curve steepness)

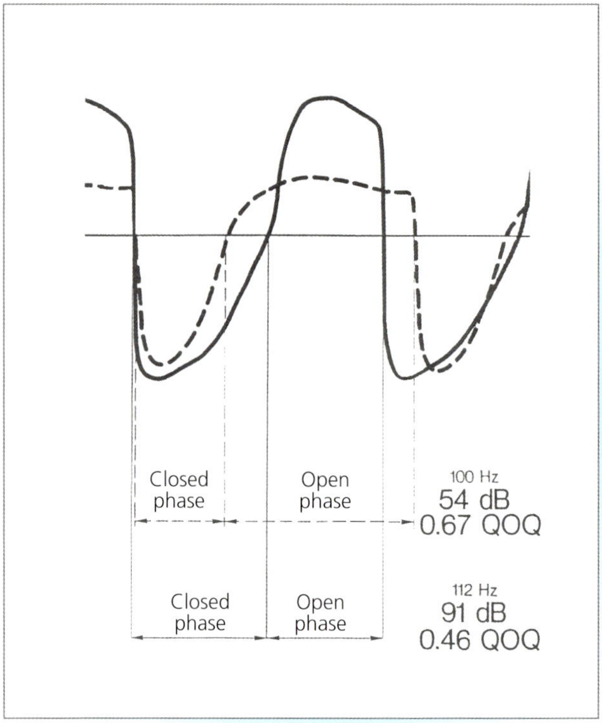

Figure 6.3
Electroglottogram in normal, soft (dotted line) and louder (solid line) phonation of a male test person with a healthy voice (Hacki, 1989a, 1989b).

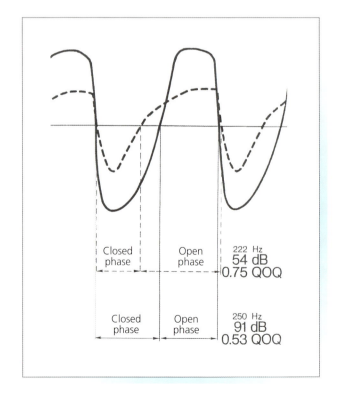

Figure 6.4
Electroglottogram in normal, soft (dotted line) and louder (solid line) phonation of a female test person with a healthy voice (Hacki, 1989a, 1989b).

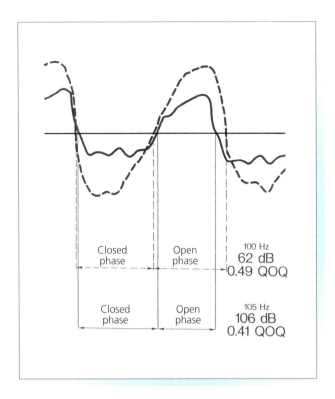

Closed phase | Open phase | 100 Hz
62 dB
0.49 QOQ

Closed phase | Open phase | 105 Hz
106 dB
0.41 QOQ

Figure 6.5
EGG of a male patient with hyperfunctional dysphonia for soft (dotted line) and loud (solid line) phonation (Hacki, 1989a, 1989b).

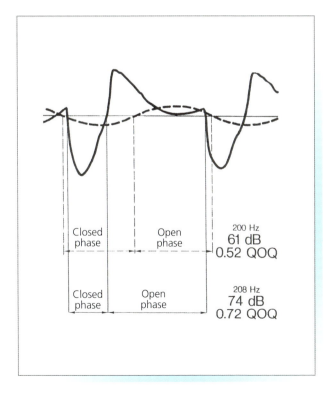

Closed phase | Open phase | 200 Hz
61 dB
0.52 QOQ

Closed phase | Open phase | 208 Hz
74 dB
0.72 QOQ

Figure 6.6
EGG of a female patient with hypofunctional dysphonia for soft (dotted line) and loud (solid line) phonation (Hacki, 1989a, 1989b).

- assessment of voice onset and build-up
- assessment of hyperfunctional and hypofunctional dysphonia
- used as a biofeedback method (e.g. Hacki, 1989a, 1989b; Kitzing, 1990).

The relationship between electroglottography and laryngeal carcinoma is described in the literature (Sopko, 1980; Orlikoff et al., 1999). Nevertheless, the diagnosis of vocal fold carcinoma cannot be done based on electroglottographic findings alone.

Information on the glottal regions located outside the vocal fold contact area during phonation may not be assessed using an electro-glottographical analysis. The opening and closing movements of the vocal folds may be registered from the outside percutaneously. This provides a very reliable basis for a fundamental frequency analysis. Therefore, some manufacturers include simultaneous displays in their stroboscopic equipment, showing the electroglottographical wave in addition to the stroboscopic vibration pattern.

Voice register and electroglottography

There is a difference in vocal fold contact during glottographical assessment of various voice registers (Figure 6.7).

Experimental examination with the aid of glottal segmentation based on electroglottography (Gall and Berg, 1998).

This involves visual assessment of the glottal cycle during repetition of the examination of the continuous changes in sound pressure within an electroglottogram. The cascading-shaped curve image shows the changing structures that are dependent on the pitch, loudness of phonation and during sound production.

Practical fact

A clinical differentiation between benign and malign laryngeal disorders is not possible by means of electroglottography (EGG). Nevertheless glottograms provide findings that contain information on vocal fold contact and glottal vibration patterns without the need for the discomfort of an endoscopic examination.

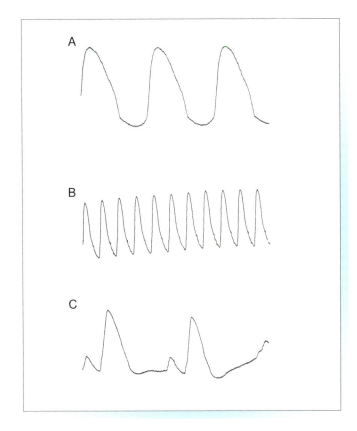

Figure 6.7
Electroglottograms of different registers
A: modal register
B: loft register
C: pulse register
(Baken, 1992).

6.4 Photoglottography (PGG) (optical glottography)

Photocell methods introduced by Sonesson in 1960 and 1962 for the analysis of vocal fold vibrations did not achieve the level of importance reached by electroglottography.

Methodology

Subglottal tissue of the throat is illuminated externally. Depending on the vibration pattern during phonation, varying amounts of light from the subglottal space reach the hypopharynx through the glottis. Here – with the help of a photocell or, more precisely, with the help of a light-sensitive transistor – the light levels are determined continuously and results are presented in the form of a curve. During this process – and after a topical anaesthesia of the laryngeal entrance if needed – a curved plexiglass probe must be inserted into the mouth to serve as an illuminating light cable. The miniaturization of transistors allows sensors also to be guided through the nose into the epipharynx.

Kitzing and Sonesson (1974) describe three quotients to be evaluated: open quotient, speed quotient and rate quotient. When pitch increases or loudness decreases, there is an increase in open quotients. The speed quotients are not influenced by loudness or pitch.

Experimental examination with the aid of strobophotoglottography (SPGG) (Hess et al., 1997, 1998)

This technique applies a stroboscopic light triggered by the fundamental frequency – in a transcutaneous manner as with photo-glottography; the light is detected transglottally using rigid video-endoscopy. Thus glottographical findings are also received in addition to video-stroboscopic sequences.

7. Ultrasound

7.1 Preliminary remarks

The term 'ultrasoundglottography' was formerly used to describe the analysis of vocal fold vibrations with the aid of ultrasound. Ultrasonic diagnostics are based on the impulse-echo principle, however. This means that the sound waves are wholly or partially reflected on the boundary surface. Since the term 'ultrasoundglottography' is thus misleading, we suggest the term 'echolaryngography' (Boehme, 1988a, 1988b, 1989, 1990, 1991, 1992 and 2000).

Historical review

The principle of ultrasonic assessment of the larynx was first described in 1964 by the Frenchman Mensch and in the same year by the Japanese team Kitamura, Kaneko and Asano. Despite various experimental formats (transmission methods with two ultrasound heads, reflection methods with a transducer, and utilization of the Doppler effect) and the efforts of various groups (Hertz et al., 1970; Holmer et al., 1973; Kaneko et al., 1983; Kelsey et al., 1969; Miura, 1969; Suzuki et al., 1986; Zagzebski et al., 1983) the technique was not able to establish itself within laryngology and phoniatrics.

Examination methods of echolaryngography

Table 7.1 summarizes the special technique in ultrasound diagnostics for glottal vibration analysis with the aid of simultaneous B- and M-mode recordings, as well as the Doppler, duplex and colour-coded duplex techniques (echolaryngography).

Table 7.1 Ultrasound diagnostics of the larynx (echolaryngography): options for glottal motion and vibration analysis

• *Two-dimensional ultrasound* B-Mode (brightness mode) M-Mode (time motion technique)	} simultaneous
• *Duplex sonography* PW Doppler (PW = pulsed wave) and B-Mode	• *Colour duplex sonography* PW Doppler and B-Mode and Colour coding

Figure 7.1

Echolaryngography: Sections (Boehme, 1988a, 1988b).

1–4 transversal
5   medio-sagittal
6   coronary

1–4 transversal sections
- subglottal level
- thyroid cartilage level
- supraglottis
- pre-epiglottal level

5–6 vertical levels (medio-sagittal, coronary)
- pre-epiglottal level
- vocal fold-false vocal fold level

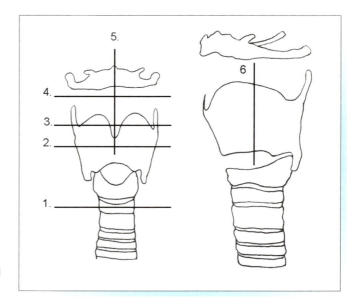

The transcutaneous approaches can be divided into (1) transversal and (2) vertical sections. Individual sections are easily identified from the above diagram (Figure 7.1a and b).

7.2   B-Mode and simultaneous B-M-Mode for glottal imaging

Transversal assessment of the glottis using B-Scan techniques provides an overview of the vocal fold structures during phonation and respiration (Figure 7.2). Representation of the vocal fold, or rather the false vocal fold complex, can never be achieved consistently during routine examination. Usually, *double-sided* ultrasonic diagnostics of the vocal folds is possible.

Figure 7.2

Ultrasound diagnostics at the glottal level. Vocal fold – false vocal fold complex. Respiration, B-mode, transversal.

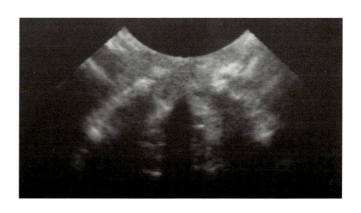

Schade and Kothe (1999) applied high-resolution B-scan echography in harmonic tissue imaging mode and selected the ligamentum conicum for transmission into the larynx. This enables visualization of the endolaryngeal conditions. If necessary, the glottis can also be assessed by positioning the transducer at the upper margin of the thyroid cartilage and directing transmission dorsally and slightly caudally (Uttenweiler, 2000). Zappia and Campani (2000) performed a morphological and functional transcutaneous ultrasound examination of the larynx in 50 healthy subjects (30 women, 20 men, age: up to 74 years), 17 of whom were professional opera singers. The subjects were examined in a supine position with the neck overextended. The authors were able to differentiate intralaryngeal structures with the aid of a 7.5 MHz scanner by applying an anterior-posterior and caudocranial ray path. They also measured the length and thickness of the vocal folds of both females and males.

Coronary assessment of the glottis by simultaneous B- and M-mode ultrasound imaging is a promising method for analysing motion and vibration of the glottis. Coronary assessment involves *unilateral imaging of the vocal fold.*

Motion analysis of the vocal fold with the aid of M-mode echo amplitudes provides information about tissue properties with different motion amplitudes. More or less pronounced echo amplitudes, as well as echo transmission times in M-mode can be recognized when the measuring line is guided through the moving vocal fold during phonation in B-mode (Figure 7.3).

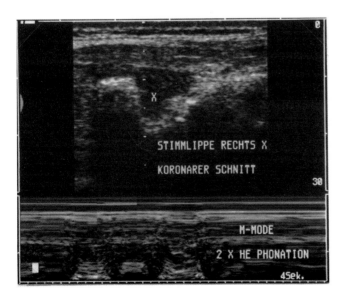

Figure 7.3
Movement analysis of the right vocal fold. Simultaneous B- and M-mode, coronary.
Upper part: Line of measurement moves through vocal fold (B-mode).
Lower part: 2x /he/ phonation (M-mode).

Figure 7.4
Vibration analysis of the right vocal fold simultaneously in B- and M-mode. Coronary.
Upper half of the image: B-mode coronary from the right. The measuring line runs through the vibrating vocal fold.
Lower half of the image: M-mode with a time window of 2 secs. M-tone phonation (approx. 75 Hz). Approx. 150 vocal fold vibrations are visualized as a vertical motion pattern.

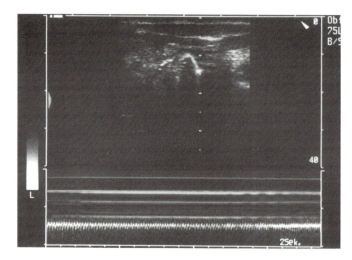

Vibration analysis of the vocal fold in M-mode enables frequency determination over a period in milliseconds. However, vibration analysis of the vocal fold can be performed only during deep phonation and (depending on the technical options available) is not always successful (Figure 7.4).

Clinical experience is reported by Uttenweiler (2000), who applies B-M-mode with colour flow to assess the pressed voice onset in dysphonia and vocal fold pareses in the course of therapy.

7.3 Duplex sonography of the glottis

Doppler sonography of the larynx was introduced as a diagnostic procedure as early as 1968 (Minifie et al.). Schindler et al. (1990) applied the simultaneous B-mode and pulsating Doppler technique to assess the vibration velocity of the vocal fold. In two test subjects, and one patient with unilateral vocal fold paralysis, he succeeded in

Practical fact

Simultaneous B- and M-mode imaging for the motion and vibration analysis of the glottis requires further studies properly to assess its clinical value.

performing an analysis of the glottis which yielded objective physiological and pathological findings besides involving the usual endoscopic techniques applied in vibration diagnostics of the vocal cord. We (Boehme, 1991, 1992) were able to perform a vibration analysis of the intralaryngeal structures by duplex sonography. The results obtained are discussed below.

Duplex sonography is a combination of B-mode sonography with additional pulsating Doppler. This enables flow velocity measurements in angiology. Mysonography of the vocal folds involves an analysis of flow velocities. As in the blood flow assessment, a frequency-time spectrum can now also be obtained from the measured vocal fold tissue.

Duplex sonography of the larynx is best performed at the glottal level with the aid of a transversal section plane. For this purpose, we orient ourselves on the thyroid cartilage skeleton and look for the glottis level with the aid of pulsed Doppler during /he/-phonation. A typical Doppler spectrum can be obtained in this way, even though the pocket fold structures of the voice folds are not observed during phonation. This is a frequency analysis with a *frequency-time spectrum*. The Doppler spectrum contains a number of different frequencies and intensities.

Methodology

A pulsed Doppler is used. The Doppler shift – that is, the positive and negative amplitudes of the Doppler spectrum – depends on the direction of movement of the intralaryngeal structures, especially the vocal folds. If the moving reflection surface comes closer to the Doppler probe, a positive Doppler shift will occur; if the reflection surface moves away from the Doppler probe, a negative Doppler shift occurs. The simultaneous appearance of the current B-image in addition to the Doppler signal allows for an easier examination process. The glottal level may be adjusted at the transversal section. Even if no morphological structures at the glottal level can be found in the B-scan, a Doppler ultrasound of the glottis can be taken using a precise transversal image section technique. The examination may be limited to special vocal fold regions. We used a frequency filtering below 100Hz and above 2000Hz.

For this purpose a *sample volume* is used. The selected tissue volume may be adjusted into various lengths using the sample volume. We selected a sample volume 2–4 mm in length and positioned it in the vocal fold region. If needed, the entire vocal fold pattern may be tested using the Doppler mode.

Normal findings

Figure 7.5 shows a transversal section at the glottal level with the thyroid cartilage identified. Intralaryngeal details do not appear in this B-image representation. The sample volume is adjusted in the middle of the assumed glottal area. Given the length in millimetres as determined above, the desired glottal structure of this region may be targeted and assessed. If using /he/ phonation, a pulsed Doppler spectrum of this region now may be made. The pulsed Doppler spectrum corresponds to the phonation time (Figure 7.5, left side). The Doppler spectrum may be explained as follows.

Figure 7.5
Duplex sonography of the larynx in the glottal area (a) and supraglottis (b) during /he/ phonation. Horizontal section, pulsed Doppler.

(a) Doppler spectrum present in B-image, sample volume at the level of non-visible vocal folds.

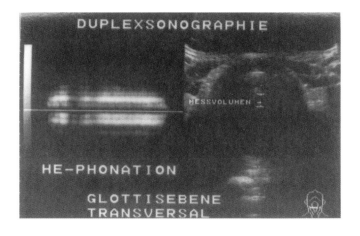

(b) Doppler spectrum not in evidence, since the sample volume in the B-image is located outside the glottis (supraglottal).

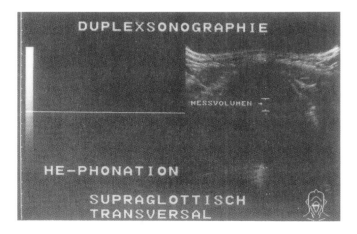

When the moving glottis comes closer to the Doppler probe, a positive Doppler shift occurs; when the glottis moves away from the Doppler probe, then a negative Doppler shift occurs. These two components determine the curve configuration above and below the zero line within the Doppler spectrum.

If the sample volume moves away from the vibrating glottal level, and moves to a supraglottal level during a transversal B-scan examination with the sound head for example, the Doppler spectrum is no longer visible (Figure 7.5b, left side). Doppler testing cannot be performed to show sample volumes in the air-filled supraglottal portion.

During crescendo and decrescendo phonation with pitch variations, formants may be identified during /he/ phonation (Figure 7.6).

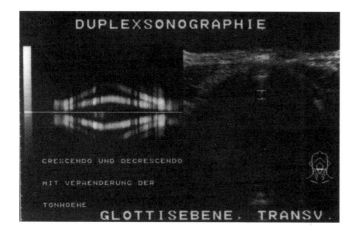

Figure 7.6
Duplex sonography of the larynx in the glottal level. Horizontal section, pulsed Doppler. Crescendo and decrescendo with change in pitch.

Clinical application

In cases of inflammation or paralysis within the laryngeal region, there will be a very different pulsed Doppler spectrum for the glottis. When a comparison is made between a compensated left vocal fold paralysis with glottal closure during phonation (Figure 7.7a) with a decompensated flaccid left vocal fold paralysis without glottal closure during phonation (Figure 7.7b), strongly varying Doppler spectrums will occur. Now a clear time-shifted positive and negative Doppler shift may be identified. Simultaneously during /he/ phonation, a prominent aperiodicity in the Doppler spectrum takes place. The more dysphonic a patient is, the more the structures in the Doppler spectrum are lost.

Figure 7.7
Duplex sonography in the glottal level. Horizontal section, pulsed Doppler.

(a) Rigid (compensated) left vocal fold paralysis: not in evidence in the B-image glottal structures. Tuning curve with sample volume is median. Light aperiodicity within the Doppler spectrum, prominent at the end of /he/ phonation.

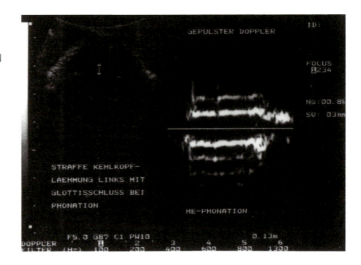

(b) Flaccid (decompensated) left vocal fold paralysis: not in evidence in the B-image glottal structures. Tuning curve with sample volume is located laterally on the (non-visible) left paresis vocal cord. During /he/ phonation there is strong aperiodicity within the Doppler spectrum.

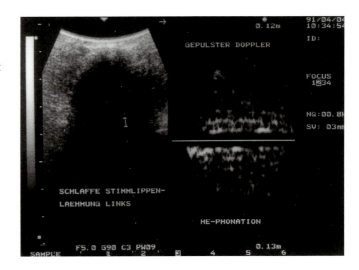

Practical fact

Duplex sonography of the glottis improves the sensitivity of B-image laryngeal sonography, and thus improves the accuracy of vibration analysis of the vocal fold motion cycle. The duplex examination of the glottis enriches our knowledge of the sonophysiology of the larynx. There is a lack of clinical experience regarding glottal vibration ability performed using duplex sonography. Thus other procedures, such as stroboscopy, high-speed cinematography, and videokymography lead to much more informative results.

7.4   Colour-coded duplex sonography of the glottis

Colour-coded duplex sonography of the larynx may be undertaken using a combined application of B-image sonography, pulsed Doppler testing and colour coding. During phonation, a coloured representation of moving intralaryngeal structures is made when the entire larynx is examined in a colour mode with *transversal section* (Boehme, 1991, 1992).

By assigning various colours, the direction of motions and motion speed of intralaryngeal portions may be recorded. In duplex mode, a detailed analysis of the peripheral structures of surrounding intralaryngeal portions may be performed using spectral analysis with a pulsed Doppler technique.

Colour-coded duplex sonography depends on:

- the fundamental frequency of the voice, and
- the motion speed (adjustment of equipment required).

Intralaryngeal motions towards the probe are red-coded; motions away from the probe are blue-coded. Given an increase in speed, red colours turn yellow, and dark blue becomes light blue or green.

Normal findings

During /he/ phonation it is possible to see the same motions for each side of intralaryngeal structures, including the glottis, or even all intralaryngeal portions depending on the speed of motion. Thus it again becomes clear that all intralaryngeal structures may be included during phonation. As may be identified in Figure 7.8, the median glottal sections tend to vibrate more. In contrast, all intralaryngeal structures may be included in the vibration process (Figure 7.9).

Practical fact

Using this technique, a vibration analysis of vocal folds for the entire intralaryngeal tissue is possible.

Figure 7.8
Colour-coded duplex sonography of the larynx.
Normal findings: Transversal section at glottal level. Measurement range of motion speed 0–92 cm/s.
Red coloured: Motion pattern towards Doppler probe.
Blue coloured: Motion pattern away from Doppler probe.

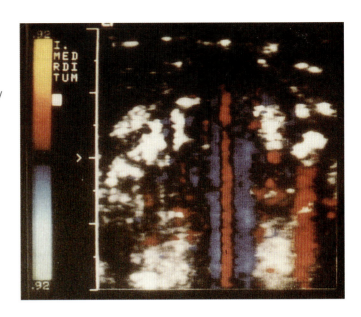

Figure 7.9
Colour-coded duplex sonography of the larynx.
Normal findings: Transversal section at glottal level. Measurement range of motion speed 0–34 cm/s.
Red coloured: Motion pattern towards Doppler probe.
Blue coloured: Motion pattern away from Doppler probe.

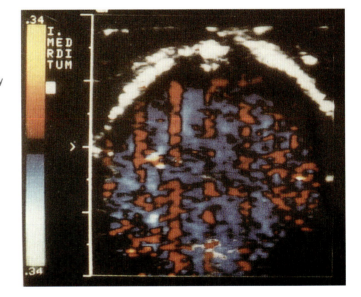

Clinical applications

Colour-coded duplex sonography of the larynx indicates a varying colour code in the case of a *left-side rigid (compensated) vocal fold paralysis* between the right and left halves of the larynx (Figure 7.10).

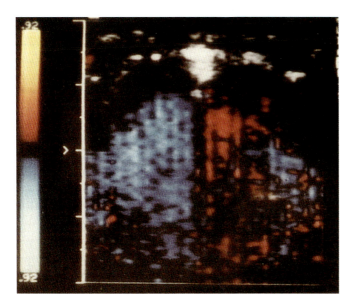

Figure 7.10
Colour-coded duplex sonography of the larynx. Left vocal fold paralysis. Transversal section at glottal level. Measurement range of motion speed 0–92 cm/s.
Red coloured: Motion pattern towards Doppler probe.
Blue coloured: Motion pattern away from Doppler probe.

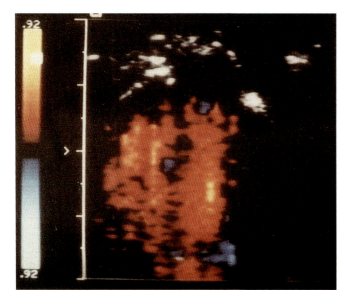

Figure 7.11
Colour-coded duplex sonography of the larynx. Laryngeal carcinoma T4 on left side. Transversal section at glottal level. Measurement range of motion speed 0–92 cm/s.
Red coloured: Motion pattern towards Doppler probe.
Blue coloured: Motion pattern away from Doppler probe.

During /he/ phonation the healthy right side of the larynx almost always moves away from the Doppler probe; thus a blue colour code appears. In contrast, during /he/ phonation the left paresis vocal fold moves both towards and away from the Doppler probe. Thus the colour code is partly red and partly blue.

Practical fact

The functional analysis of one-sided vocal fold paralysis using duplex sonography indicates that despite vibratory immobility, there is a pathological vibration mechanism of the vocal fold tissue on the paralysed side. This correspond to the laryngostroboscopic findings.

In the case of *laryngeal carcinoma* on the left side of the larynx a colour coding is not in evidence (Figure 7.11). The reason is a fixation of the tumour on the left so that motion patterns do not occur during respiration or during phonation. As a result, with the help of pulsed Doppler technique there is no motion towards or away from the Doppler probe – thus the left side cannot be assigned a colour code. Apparently the size of the infiltrating tumour of the glottal region plays a decisive role. During recent tests performed involving T1 glottal tumours, no pathological findings were in evidence using colour-coded duplex sononography.

Ooi et al. (1995) confirmed these vibration analyses of the glottis by means of colour coded duplex sonography in 10 normal people and eight patients with dysphonia. They also reported the findings obtained in three patients with unilateral vocal fold paralysis.

Practical fact

Colour-coded duplex sonography of the glottis and the intralaryngeal region is technically complicated. Its future application in laryngology and phoniatrics is possible. However, further studies are required to gain more extensive knowledge about this type of vibration analysis of the glottis. In the meantime, other procedures like stroboscopy and imaging techniques like MRI and CT will prevail for daily routine use.

7.5   The situation after laryngectomy

Assessment of the pharyngo-oesophageal segment after a laryngectomy (with and without voice prosthesis) with the help of ultrasonic ultrasound diagnosis (7.5 resp. 5 MHz transducer) in B- and M-mode provide a good overview of:

• differentiated morphological structures (B-mode), and
• differentiated vibration pattern of the pseudoglottis (M-mode)

for people who are good oesophageal speakers (Boehme, 1988a, 1988b). When speaking, an echo-rich ring structure in B-mode is formed in the area of the pharyngo-oesophagal segment in the transversal section. This represents the pseudo-glottis. Figures 7.12a and b illustrate the good differentiation between the pharyngo-esophageal segment (B-mode) and the excellent structure of the echo amplitudes in M-mode in a laryngectomee. This may be identified easily in a spoken phrase.

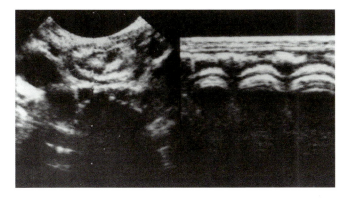

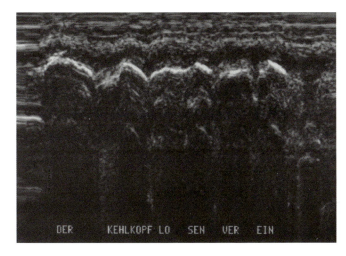

Figure 7.12
Laryngectomee (58 years) with good oesophageal voice. Echomorphological and functional features during repeated /0/ phonation. B- and M-mode. Simultaneous imaging. Transversal section. At the level of the measurement line (B-mode) there is evidence of good function for the pharyngo-oesophagal segment (M-mode). M-mode, transversal in the middle of the pharyngeo-oesophageal segment. The functional result of a good speaker is proved by a structured representation of the test phrase 'Der Kehlkopflosenverein'.

(a) top
B- and M-mode simultaneously.
(b) bottom
M-mode.

Practical fact

The analysis of movements and vibrations of the pharyngo-oesophageal segment after laryngectomy with the help of B- and M-mode may be accepted as a routine method.

8. Kymography

Prior to the first application of kymography on the larynx, the technique had been proven already in other topics. For example, in recording heart motions, registration of pupil movement, and depiction of the flow of corpuscular blood in capillaries. Given encouragement by Pfau, Gall et al. developed a new method for photokymographical examination of the vibratory cycle of vocal folds in 1971.

8.1 Techniques

8.1.1 Photokymography

Four basic methods are possible for photokymographical recording of laryngeal movements: area, stripe, raster, and step photokymography as a modification of stripe photokymography.

Area photokymography
This technique is based on a specially modified slit shutter. This shutter, with a constant width of approximately 0.5–0.8 mm, moves from one edge of the image to the other at a constant speed. A sequence of line-shaped images of the object is thus formed. If the slit shutter moves, e.g. perpendicular to the vocal fold vibration axis, the image will be distorted depending on the amplitude and frequency. Thus an image results in which all phases of directly consecutive vibrations may be seen (Figure 8.1). The advantage of this method is that when recording all non-moving object sections, as with a normal photo, morphology can be assessed and all moving sections with all consecutive vibration phases may be presented together within one image (Figure 8.2).

Gall et al. (1971), Gall and Hanson (1973), Gall and Freigang (1974) and Gall (1978) used area photokymography to present findings from organic and functional laryngeal disorders. The continuous depiction with vibrating vocal folds and juxtaposition of all vibration phases within one image provided not only photographic documentation of the glottal findings, but at the same time provided the basis for determining many physical parameters (duration of vibration period, open phase, closed phase, open quotient, opening speed, speed quotient, length of vocal folds, false vocal fold distance). In contrast, using stroboscopy and cinematography, these parameters

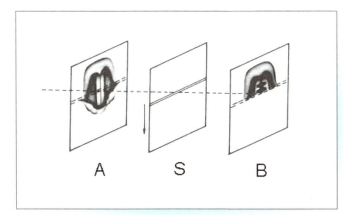

Figure 8.1
Diagram of area photokymography according to Gross.
A = laryngoscopic image as normally seen using a laryngeal mirror or rigid endoscope.
S = directly in front of a light-sensitive film a slit shutter is located perpendicular to the vocal fold vibration axis, from the top to bottom of image edge.
B = area photokymogram.

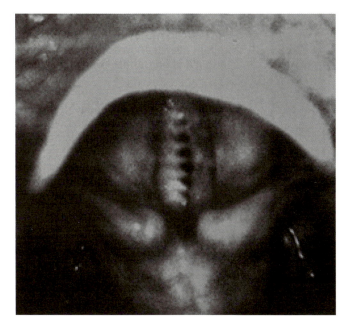

Figure 8.2
Area photokymography of inflammation of the left vocal fold after polyp removal. Incomplete glottal closure, periodic vibrations, asymmetry of amplitudes (left < right), no major phase shifts, no phonatoric immobility.

could be achieved only with intricate assessment of several continuous images (Gall and Hanson, 1973).

Stripe photokymography

In contrast to the area method, stripe photokymography involves a lined-shaped image frame released by a slit shutter whereby the film is moved at a constant speed. In this way vibrations in the area of the line-shaped image frame are photographed consecutively and kept within one image (Figure 8.3). The advantage of this technique is that the vibration process is photographed continuously as one and the same anatomical structure. The disadvantage is that only a small line of the entire larynx is displayed; thus the anatomical structure being tested cannot be identified based on the image. Anatomical details on the surrounding regions are thus not depicted (Figure 8.4). To record the function of the entire glottis, a successive sampling from the anterior to posterior is required. The aim is that phonation should remain constant for all samples taken during partial assessments.

Figure 8.3
Diagram of stripe photokymography according to Gross (1988).
A = laryngoscopic image as normally seen in a laryngeal mirror or using rigid endoscope.
S = directly behind the fixed slit shutter, a light-sensitive film is moved perpendicular to the vocal fold vibration axis.
B = Stripe photokymogram.

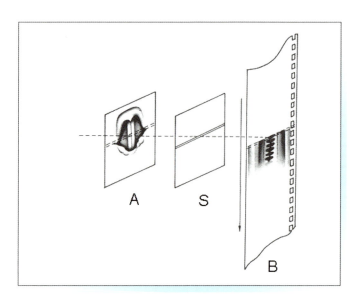

Figure 8.4
Stripe photokymography of a patient with an inflammation of the left vocal fold.
Glottal closure: complete
Amplitude: right normal, left reduced
Symmetry: amplitudes asymmetric without marked phase shift
Periodicity: periodic
Regularity: normal vibration mode
Mucosal wave: right normal, left reduced
Phonatory immobility: not present
Supraglottic constriction: not assessable

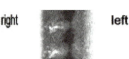
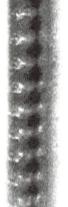

The problems surrounding stripe photokymography appear relatively simple to solve technically (Gall, 1984a); Gross (1988) introduced a specially adapted test unit Type F III from the manufacturer ROBOT.

Area kymograms of the glottis were first presented by Gall et al., in 1971. Between 1980 and 1988 Gross further developed kymography for application using an endoscope and for semi-automatic digital assessment with more than 400 parameters.

Videokymography

Videokymography is the logical development following photo stripe kymography, whereby a single line is exposed to a CCD camera with up to 8000 images per second (Figure 8.5). Due to its high level of light-sensitivity and simple preparation, videokymography has many clear advantages over photokymography. Building on the preliminary investigations of Švec and Schutte (1996), Schutte, Švec and Šram (1998) reported clinical results that indicate a possible optimization of analysis options in contrast to stroboscopy.

Unlike videostroboscopy, videokymography does not provide an overview of the larynx. The limitations of laryngeal stroboscopy may be overcome using videokymography. This applies, for example, to:

- poor voice quality with lack of stroboscopic triggering, and
- aperiodicity of vocal fold vibrations.

In fact, this method provides considerably more details of vibration patterns than does stroboscopy. The findings of Gall and Gross also

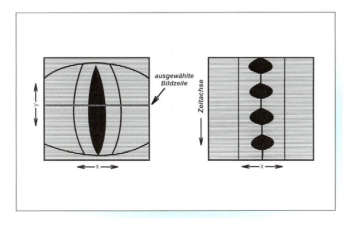

Figure 8.5

Two methods using a videokymography camera. On the left a standard mode for vocal fold imaging is used. The entire picture consists of horizontal lines. In high-speed kymography mode the camera can select a single line to record vocal fold motions. The resulting videokymographic image is seen on the left. The vertical axis corresponds to the time. Adapted from Švec and Schutte (1996).

confirm that many more deviations from an ideal vibration mode exist in the case of a normal voice than may be seen in the results of stroboscopic and high-speed cinematographic recordings. Figures 8.6 to 8.11 demonstrate the details provided for various voice disorders (e.g. Švec and Šram , 1998 and Dejonckere, 2000).

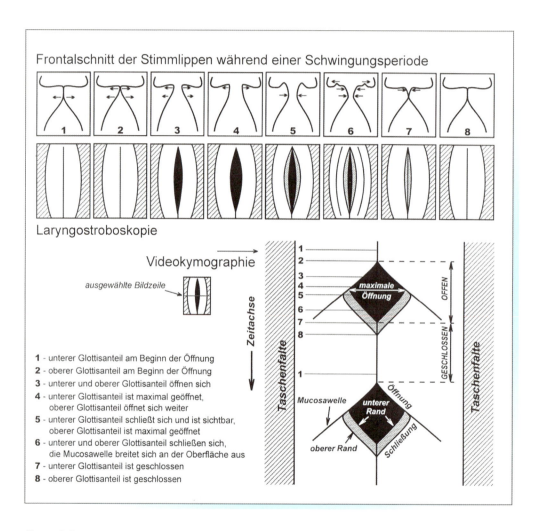

Figure 8.6

Diagram of features of normal vocal fold vibration in comparison to laryngostroboscopy and videokymography. Adapted from Švec, Šram and Schutte (1999).

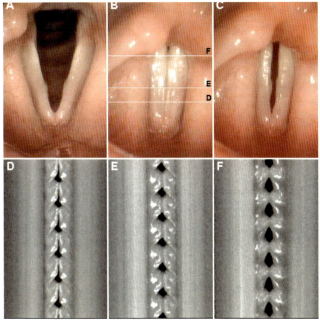
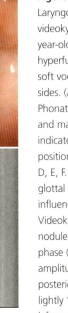

Figure 8.7
Laryngoscopic, stroboscopic and videokymographic images of a 24-year-old female patient with hyperfunctional dysphonia and soft vocal fold nodules on both sides. (A) Respiration. (B) and (C) Phonation with maximum closure and maximum opening. The lines indicate the measurement positions of the videokymograms D, E, F. (D) Vibration in anterior glottal section. Closed phase is influenced by the nodules. (E) Videokymogram at vocal fold nodule level. Prolonged closed phase (CQ = ca. 0.7) and reduced amplitude. (F) Vibration in posterior glottal section. The lightly 'rippled' movement of the left vocal fold during the open phase indicates impaired vibration behaviour. Fundamental frequency of the voice is about 320 Hz, total duration of recording about 18 ms for all videokymograms (Šram and Švec, 2000).

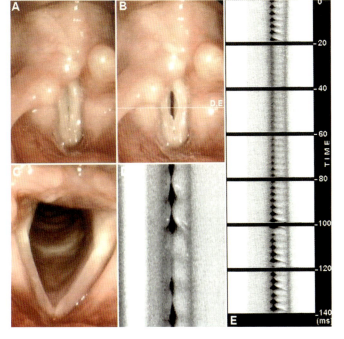

Figure 8.8
Laryngoscopic, stroboscopic and videokymographic images of a 53-year-old female patient with spasmodic adductor type dysphonia. (A) and (B) Phonation with maximum closure and maximum opening. (C) Respiration. (D) Videokymogram in the position marked in (B) (total duration of recording about 18 ms). Sequence of juxtaposed videokymographical images (Šram and Švec, 2000).

Figure 8.9

Videokymograms illustrating the variability of phonation in the case of spasmodic adductor type dysphonia (same patient as in Figure 8.8). The recording position was similar to that of Fig. 8.8B. Total duration of recording ca. 18 ms for all videokymograms (Šram and Švec, 2000).

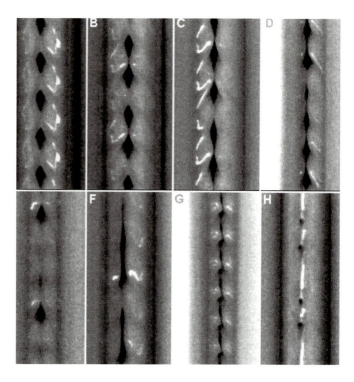

Figure 8.10

Laryngoscopic, stroboscopic and videokymographic images of a 29-year-old female patient with one-sided vocal fold paralysis on the right. (A) Phonation with maximally-closed glottis. (B) Phonation with maximally-opened glottis. Horizontal lines indicate the measurement position of the videokymogram. (C) Respiration (D) Videokymographic details of the vibration pattern of both vocal folds. Total duration of recording ca. 18 ms. (E) sequence of consecutive videokymograms reveals changes of vibration pattern over a total time frame of 140 ms. The slight bulge in the vibration pattern is caused by the patient's or the endoscope's motion during examination (Šram, Švec and Schutte, 1999).

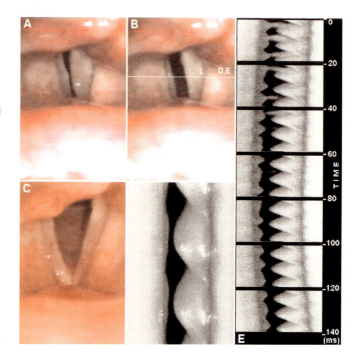

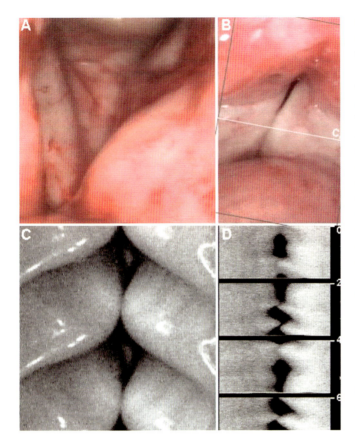

Figure 8.11
Laryngoscopic, stroboscopic and videokymographic images of a 69-year-old female patient with a false vocal fold phonation as a result of a right chordectomy ten years before. **(A)** Respiration. **(B)** Adducted false vocal folds during phonation. The horizontal line indicates the measurement position of the videokymograms C and D (the video camera is slightly rotated in order to adjust the measurement line to a position nearly perpendicular to the pseudoglottis). **(C)** Videokymogram of a false vocal fold phonation with good voice quality: fundamental frequency ca. 120 Hz, large vibration amplitudes, prominent mucosal waves (total duration of recording ca. 18 ms).
(D) Consecutive videokymograms of false vocal fold phonation with a slightly worse (hoarser) voice quality: irregular vibrations of false vocal folds with small amplitudes (Šram, Švec and Schutte, 1999).

Practical fact

Diagnosis of organic and functional voice disorders with the help of videokymography delivers a host of details by way of a line-shaped image; this is well-suited for quantitative assessment purposes. In contrast to stroboscopy, videokymography reveals many more visible distinctive features of vocal fold vibration pattern even in cases of normal voice production.

8.1.3 High speed kymography

This technique automatically extracts kymograms of vocal fold vibrations from digital high-speed recordings (see also high-speed cinematography, Chapter 9). This allows calculation of parameters such as location/time diagrams, fundamental frequency, open and closed quotients, oscillation time, jitter and shimmer. Wittenberg et al. (1998) use a new kymographic technique for high-speed recordings which combines the two recording media described above. With the help of digital image processing, kymograms may be extracted and automatically evaluated from recordings made by digital high-speed cameras.

8.1.4 Videostrobokymography

Previously recorded and digitally saved videostroboscopic sequences were reworked kymographically by Myung-Whun Sung et al. in 1999. By combining a line from each individual image in a series, kymograms were created which could be digitally and quantitatively analysed. This technique is inferior to high-speed kymography, however.

9. High-speed cinematography

An assessment of vocal fold vibrations based on high-speed cinematography was first performed by Farnsworth (1940). Investigations by Timcke et al. (1959), Leden et al. (1960) and Leden and Moore (1961) fundamentally expanded our knowledge.

The most important advantage of high-speed cinematography is the large time resolution. Only with this considerable resolution it is possible to observe normal and pathological vibration patterns. High-speed cinematography fulfils the requirements of Shannon's sampling theory, which indicates that the sampling rate must be two times higher than the vocal fold fundamental frequency (f_0). Due to the short-term variability of fundamental frequency (jitter) and amplitude (shimmer), oversampling also is needed primarily with a factor of between $5f_0$ and $10f_0$ during clinical recording.

From an historical perspective (Köster, 1997) two phases in the development of high-speed cinematography may be identified:

- mechanical or analogue high-speed cinematography, and
- digital high-speed cinematography.

9.1   Mechanical high-speed cinematography

Although mechanical high-speed cinematography has influenced voice physiology and voice pathology decisively regarding vocal fold vibration analysis, the various techniques remain only historically meaningful from today's perspective. Given problems in managing

Practical fact

In principle, high-speed cinematography provides much information during analysis of vocal fold vibrations. In contrast to videokymography, analysis using high-speed cinematography requires additional evaluation software with automatic signal recognition. Due to its high cost, the techniques have not yet developed into routine methods.

insufficient lighting, heat development, noise strain and time-consuming individual image evaluation, mechanical high-speed cinematography has been excluded from many laboratory applications. Once analogue techniques were replaced by digital high-speed cinematography in the 1980s, opportunities arose for high-speed cinematography methods.

9.2   Digital high-speed cinematography

The advantages of digital high-speed cinematography are obvious: for example, digital image sequences may be called up immediately and directly. In comparison with analogue and other analytic methods, digital high-speed cinematography has a host of advantages: Recordings are available directly and may be checked for quality and information represented. By combining with night vision equipment, which illuminates by a factor of 1500, recordings may also be made using light sources and endoscopes with weak light, e.g. with a flexible rhinolaryngoscope. The image frequency is variable for several systems, so that the optimal setting may be chosen depending on the nature of the task according to Shannon's sampling theory. Since information is already available in digital form, it may be used for an automatic digital assessment without undergoing an additional conversion process. There are several systems available for digital high-speed cinematography, which differ in picture resolution, frame rate, time needed to record each sequence, archiving, data channels, night vision equipment and colour representation (Table 9.1).

9.2.1 Motion analysis techniques

In contrast to the past when only manual methods were available, today automatic analytic systems are being used increasingly. Speed of evaluation has been increased from a maximum of 400 images/hour to 60 images/second.

Application of functional imaging is currently favoured (Spiesberger and Tasto, 1981). This technique describes the time-related motion pattern of the vocal folds at a point that may be freely chosen. Through extraction and linking all image lines with the same line index and a sequence's tilting angle, a two-dimensional image is created, described as a *digital kymogram* (Figures 9.1 and 9.2) – in much the same way as during videokymography (Wittenberg).

Table 9.1 Comparison of digital high-speed cinematography systems for examination of human phonation

Type of camera		Camsys+ 128	Camsys+ 256	Self-manufactured RILP	Kodak EktaPro	Kodak 1000 HRC
Maximal resolution	[Pixel²]	128 x 128	256 x 256	128 x 32	200 x 240	640 x 480
Standard recording rate	[Hz]	2000	500	2500	1000	250
Maximal recording rate	[Hz]	10000	3700	2500	6000	1000
Standard length of time to record	[Sec]	8.1	8.1	6	2.4	2
		Digital		Digital	Video	
Options: data channels		2		2	1	1
		EGG, audio possible		EGG, audio	Audio	Audio
night vision equipment		No		No	Yes	No
colour				No	No	Yes

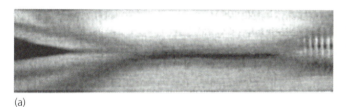

(a)

(b)

(c)

Figure 9.1
Digital videokymograms of different voice onsets (turned 90°); left: transition from respiration to phonation. In the hard voice onset the vocal folds are pressed together prior to phonation, in the breathy voice onset the vocal folds are positioned tightly together and touch each other during vocal fold vibration (Wittenberg, 1998).

(a) hard voice onset
(b) normal voice onset
(c) breathy voice onset

Digital high-speed cinematography for vocal fold vibration analysis has not become a routine technique and is applied in individual research centres for experimental purposes only. Below is a short summary of the results of selected work groups (see also Köster, 1997).

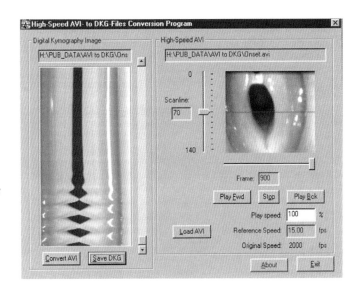

Figure 9.2
Digital videokymography: screen of a commercial digital videokymography unit in combination with high-speed cinematography (Kay Elemetrics Corporation).
Left side: videokymogram, right side: high-speed cinematography with position marked where vibration analysis is actually performed.

Kay Elemetrics System (New Jersey, USA)

The high-speed system of the Kay Elemetrics Corporation is based on the combination of videokymography and high-speed cinematography of the vocal folds. It captures at a rate of 2000 frames/sec. The system is the first one available for this purpose (Figure 9.2).

The Berlin System

Since 1993, examination has been possible with the aid of digital high-speed cinematography (Hess and Gross, 1993; Hess et al., 1996; Maurer et al., 1996). Two different Kodak camera systems offer a recording rate of (a) up to 12,000 images per second in black and white and (b) 2000 images in colour recorded digitally (Figure 9.3). Rigid endoscopy, flexible laryngoscopy and microscopes serve as optical systems. The number of image lines and/or image sections depends on time resolution; the number becomes smaller the more images are recorded per unit of time. Within this system, lighting is of only secondary importance, since a highly effective night vision system is already present. In part, it was proven that phonatoric and pre- and post-phonatoric vocal fold vibrations (which cannot be evaluated using stroboscopy) may be recorded perfectly at the same time. By means of additional triggering, the group was also able to make simultaneous high-speed recordings, electroglottograms and microphone signal recordings.

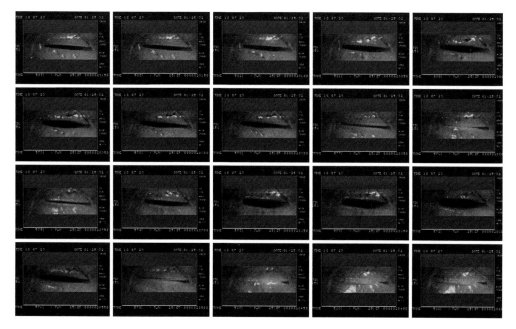

Figure 9.3
High-speed cinematographic sequence during voice onset. The closing phase is easy to see.

The Erlangen System

This group has been active since the 1980s. They developed their own digital camera system specifically for vocal fold vibration analysis (e.g. Eysholdt et al., 1996; Tigges et al., 1998; Mergell et al., 1999). In 1996 the group presented a digital high-speed camera system for laryngeal examination which reached recording speeds of up to 5600 images per second. With the help of an image processing system, all known objective parameters may be measured for voice assessment based on optical data.

In addition to a spatial resolution of 256×256 pixels and a maximal recording rate of 3700 images per second, the CAMSYS+256 system offers the longest recording time of 8.1 seconds, so that phonation is possible even during speaking, for example. By using an additional channel, the direct feeding of an EGG or acoustical signal is easily possible.

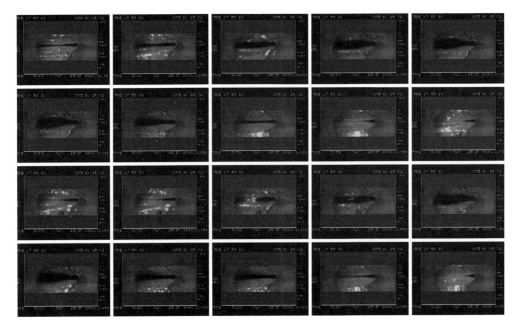

Figure 9.4

High-speed cinematographic sequence with both vocal folds in a steady state. The pictures here and in plate 9.5 are turned 90° to make optimal use of the rectangular picture cropping. The number of individual images was greatly reduced for post-processing to make the sequence of motions comprehensible.

Figure 9.5

Simultaneous depiction of a single high-speed cinematographic image (above, turned 90°), electroglottographic curve (directly beneath the image), and sound signal (second curve from the bottom). The plate shows that in the prephonatory phase, the vocal folds are already in a phonation position, while, electroglottographically, no signal has yet being formed and no voice is audible either.

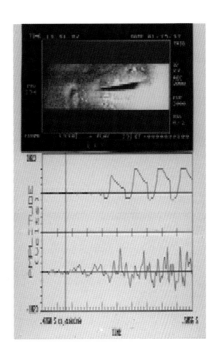

The Trier System

This system is a multimedia analysis system for digital laryngeal recordings which builds on the Berlin system (Köster, 1997). With a special video camera, the endoscope image is recorded digitally and saved digitally using a DAT recorder. The time resolution is approximately 2000 images per second with approximately 16,000 pixels per image. An electroglottographical and acoustic signal is recorded simultaneously. Data are transferred from the DAT recorder to a workstation and processed. Optical, acoustic and electro-glottographical signals are produced at the same time, resulting in a multimedia analysis system.

The Tokyo System

A detailed description and evaluation of the Japanese system, which has been undergoing further development since the mid-1980s, may be found in Köster (1997).

More recent investigations by Niimi and Miyaji (2000) using their high-speed system with 2500 images per second also include the degree of hoarseness (GRBAS scale) experienced in voice disorders in the various assessment criteria used in high-speed cinematography for pathological vocal fold vibration processes. This allows the connection of psychoacoustical evidence to objective findings.

Practical fact

High-speed recordings of vocal fold vibrations are superior in principle to stroboscopy because they do not relate to the periodicity of vibrations, and they also record vocal fold motion patterns even during initial and final transient vibration phases without phonation. In contrast to videokymography, video high-speed cinematography has the advantage of complete images with laryngomorphological presentation. A disadvantage is the evaluation software additionally required for quantitative assessment and the currently high purchasing costs involved. Yet, given the technical progress, high-speed cinematography for vocal folds still remains to be included in routine diagnostics (Hess et al., 1996).

10. Documentation

Several systems are suitable for documenting the results of vocal fold vibration analysis. These include:

- photography
- film
- video print
- video recordings
- digital recordings
- video processing.

Until now, the most common method has been video documentation, which involves using an endoscope or microscope to observe vocal fold vibrations and recording them with a video camera. The light sensitivity of such video cameras has become increasingly larger while their weight decreases. Thus video cameras are easy to handle and easy to connect to endoscopes or microscopes using adapters. Through the development of small chips, it is now possible to locate a sensor at the tip of the lens and thus further process the signal outside the patient's body.

Depending on the net frequency, in Europe video recordings with 50 half-images or 25 full images per second are largely made with the PAL video norm, while in the USA 60 half-images or 30 full images per second are made with the NTSC video norm. This image rate is sufficient to provide the human eye with a visual impression of a process of continuous motion. The combination of stroboscopy and video may produce a synchronization problem unless additional technical measures are taken. The problem arises because the stroboscope flashes do not hit the middle section of the full or half-images, but are triggered completely independently from the video-image sequence by the fundamental frequency of the vocal fold vibrations. As a result of the lack of synchronization between the stroboscope, the light and the video-image sequence, dark video images may occur – especially in contrast to the bright pictures created with multi-lighting. Various techniques may be used: photography, film, video print, video recordings, digital recordings, video preparation, multi-lighting and presentation of various vibration phases in a video image. To prevent such problems, additional synchronization between flash light and video image is required (Ludwigs et al., 1996a).

Video recordings of stroboscopic examination findings are very suitable for subsequent qualitative and quantitative assessment. If a video recorder offers the option of still imaging (jogwheel), adjustment of still images with a stroboscope, the use of a corresponding phase shift via a foot control may be completely avoided, and concentration may be focused on recording a continuous vibration sequence. With the help of video recordings, the individual vibration phases may be observed and analysed frame by frame.

Another method to document stroboscopic findings is digital recording, whereby the video signal is recorded directly on to a computer disc, where further processing may take place. With the help of corresponding software programs, subsequent processing of recordings is made easy. Deletion of failed video sequences and single images is easily possible, and labelling of single video images may be done without much effort. Mass storage should also be included when working with such digital recording methods, so that large amounts of data may be archived. By using various software programs available, retrieval is possible, e.g. according to patient name, diagnoses, recording date, etc. Back-up of previously prepared video sequences on CD-ROM, DVD or DAT is also advisable. Another recommended option is the use of a database for patient and mass back-up data.

While standard software permits further processing of digitally recorded video signals (e.g. deletion of underexposed recordings, adjustment of coloration, addition of commentary to image), special software, such as 'Dr. Speech', also allows determination of the glottal area (see Figures 5.33 and 5.34) and determination of the angles of both vocal folds to each other and in relation to the y-axis.

Practical fact

With the aid of a computer, recording, playback and archiving of audiovisual film sequences are possible. A database makes it easier to manage both patients and data.

References

Agarwal P, Bais AS (1998) A clinical and videostroboscopic evaluation of laryngeal tuberculosis. J. of Laryng. Otol. 112: 45-8.

Arens C, Glanz H, Kleinsasser O (1997) Clinical and morphological aspects of laryngeal cysts. Eur Arch Otorhinolaryngol 254: 430-6.

Arndt HJ (1994) Stimmstörungen. In P Biesalski, F Frank (eds), Phoniatrie – Pädaudiologie.Hrsg. Band 1: Phoniatrie. 2. Aufl. Stuttgart/New York: Thieme, 175–249.

Baken RJ (1992) Electroglottography. J. of Voice 6(2): 98–100.

Baken RJ, Orlikoff RF (2000) Clinical Measurement of Speech and Voice. 2nd edn. San Diego: Singular Publishing Group.

Barth V (1977) Die Lupenstroboskopie. HNO 25 (1977) 35

Bigenzahn W, Steiner E, Denk DM et al. (1998) Stroboskopie und Bildgebung in der interdisziplinären Diagnostik von Frühstadien des Larynxkarzinoms. Radiologe 38: 101–5.

Bless DM, Hicks DM (1996) Diagnosis and measurement. Assessing the 'WHs' of voice function. In WS Brown et al. (eds), Organic Voice Disorders. San Diego: Singular Publishing Group.

Bless DM, Hirano M, Feder RJ (1987) Videostroboscopy evaluation of the larynx. Ear, Nose and Throat 66: 289–96.

Boehme G (1988a) Echolaryngographie. Ein Beitrag zur Methodik der Ultraschalldiagnostik des Kehlkopfes. Laryng. Rhinol. Otol. 67: 551–8.

Boehme G (1988b) Ultraschalldiagnostik der phonatorischen Leistungen des Laryngektomierten. Laryng. Rhinol. Otol. 67: 651–6

Boehme G (1989) Ein klinischer Beitrag zur Ultraschalldiagnostik des Kehlkopfes (Echolaryngographie). Laryngo-Rhino-Otol. 68: 510–15.

Boehme G (1990) Ultraschalldiagnostik der Epiglottis. HNO 38: 355–60.

Boehme G (1991) Duplexsonographie des Kehlkopfes. 1. Bewegungsanalyse intralaryngealer Strukturen. Otorhinolaryngol Nova 1: 338–42.

Boehme G (1992) Duplexsonograpie des Kehlkopfes. 2. Farbkodierte Bewegungsanalyse intralaryngealer Strukturen. Otorhinolaryngol Nova 2: 43–5.

Boehme G (2000) Sonographie des Larynx und klinische Anwendungen (unter Ausschluss; onkologischer Erkrankungen). In R Sader, B Norer, H-H Horch (eds), Lehrbuch der Ultraschall-Diagnostik im Kopf-Halsbereich. Reinbek/Hamburg: Einhorn-Presse Verlag.

Boehme G (2003) Sprach-, Sprech-, Stimm- und Schluckstörungen. 4. Aufl. Band 1: Klinik. Munich: Urban & Fischer.

Boehme G, Gross M (2000) Phonaitrie und Paedaudiologie. Kursew für HNO-Aerzte. Berlin: Universitätsklinikum Benjamin Franklin.

Cantarella G (1998) The impact of videostroboscopy on laryngological diagnosis: a retrospective study. In: Eur Arch Oto-Rhino-Laryng. 255. Suppl. 1: 139.

Carlson E (1995) Electrolaryngography in the assessment and treatment of incomplete mutation (puberphonia) in adults. Eur. J. of Disord. of Communication 30: 140–8

Childers DG, Paige A, Moore GP (1976) Laryngeal Viteration Patterns: Arch Otolaryngol. 102: 407–10.

Colden D, Zeitels SM, Hillman RE et al. (2001) Stroboscopic assessment of vocal fold keratosis and glottic cancer. Ann Otol Rhinol Laryngol 110: 293–8.

Colton R, Casper JK (1996) Understanding Voice Problems, 2nd edn. Baltimore: Williams & Wilkins.

Cooper DM, Lawson W (1992) Laryngeal sensory receptors. In Blitzer et al. (eds), Neurologic Disorders of the Larynx. New York: Thieme.

Cornut G, Bouchayer M (1999a) Assessing Dysphonia: The Role of Videostroboscopy. An Interactive Video Textbook. Sigtuna, Sweden: The 3 Ears Company Ltd.

Cornut G, Bouchayer M (1999b) Atlas laryngostroboscopique en phonochirurgie. 10eme Cours de microchirurgie. 28–30 Jan. Lyon.

Courey MS, Garett CG, Ossoff RH (1997) Medial microflap for excision of benign vocal fold lesions. Laryngoscope 107: 340–4.

Dejonckere PH et al. (1998) Quantitative rating of videolaryngostroboscopy: a reliability study. Rev Laryngol Otol Rhinol (Bord) 119(4): 259–60.

Duncker E, Schlosshauer B (1961) Unregelmässige Stimmlippenschwingungen bei funktionellen Stimmstörungen. Z. Laryng. Rhinol. 40: 919–34.

Dursun G, Sataloff RT, Spiegel R et al. (1996) Superior laryngeal nerve paresis and paralysis. J. of Voice 10(2): 206–11.

Dworkin JP et al. (1999) Phonation subsystem outcomes following radiation therapy for T1 glottic carcinoma: a prospective voice laboratory investigation. J. Medical Speech-Language Pathology 7(3): 181–93.

Elias ME, Sataloff R Th, Rosen DC et al. (1997) Normal strobovideolaryngoscopy: variability in healthy singers. J. of Voice 11: 104–7.

Eysholdt U et al. (1996) Direct evaluation of high-speed recordings vocal fold vibrations. Folia Phoniatr Logop 48: 163–70.

Fabre P (1957) Un procédé électrique percutané d'inscription d'accolement glottique au cours de la phonation glottographie haute fréquence. Premiers résultats. Bulletin de l'Academie Nationale de Médicine 141: 66–9.

Farnsworth DW (1940) High-speed motion pictures of human vocal cords. Bell Telephone Records 18: 203–20.

Fex S (1970) Judging the movements of vocal cords in larynx paralysis. Acta Otolaryngol 263: 82–3.

Fleischer S, Hess M, Ludwigs M (1995) Die Bedeutung des Perspektivenfehlers für die Lupenlaryngoskopie, In M. Gross: Aktuelle phoniatrisch-pädaudiologische Aspekte 1994. Berlin: RGV, 105–6.

Ford CN, Bless DM (eds) (1991) Phonosurgery. New York: Raven Press.

Friedrich G (1996) Qualitätssicherung in der Phoniatrie. HNO 44: 401–16.

Friedrich G, Lichtenegger R (1997) Surgical anatomy of the larynx: J. of. Voice 11(3): 345–55.

Friedrich G, Kainz J, Freidl W (1993) Zur funktionellen Struktur der menschlichen Vocal folds. Laryngo-Rhino-Otol. 72: 215–24.

Fröhlich M, Michaelis D, Strube HW, Kruse E (1999) Akustische Stimmqualität unter verschiedenen Rahmenbedingungen. In M Gross (ed.), Aktuelle phoniatrisch-pädaudiologische Aspekte. Band 6. Heidelberg: Median-Verlag, 35–9.

Fröschels E (1937) Gesetzmässigkeiten in der Erscheinung und Entwicklung der hyperfunktionellen Heiserkeiten Mschr. f. Ohrenheilk. 71: 400–6.

Fujimura O (1981) Body-cover theory of the vocal fold and its phonetics implications. In K Steveebs, Hirano (eds), Vocal Fold Physiology. Tokyo: University of Tokyo Press, 271–81.

Gall V (1978) Fotokymographische Befunde bei funktionellen Dysphonien, Kehlkopflähmungen und Stimmlippentumoren. Folia phoniat 30: 28–35.

Gall V (1984a) Glottis-Kymographie. Habil; Holle (Jaek).

Gall V (1984b) Strip kymography of the glottis. Arch. Otorhinolaryngol 240: 287–93.

Gall V, Berg R (1998) Feinstrukturen von Stimme und Sprache. Frankfurt am Main: Edition Wötzel.

Gall V, Freigang C (1974) Zur Larynx-Fotokymographie: Demonstration einiger pathologischer Kehlkopf-Befunde. Mschr Ohr Heilk 108: 114–22.

Gall V, Hanson J (1973) Bestimmung physikalischer Parameter der Stimmlippenschwingungen mit Hilfe der Larynxphotokymographie. Folia phoniat 25: 450–9.

Gall V, Gall D, Hanson J (1971) Larynx-Fotokymografie. Arch.klin.exp. Ohr.-, Nas.-u.Kehlk.Heilk. 200: 34–41.

Gould WJ., Sataloff RTh, Spiegel JR (1993) Voice Surgery. St Louis: Mosby.

Gross M (1988) Endoskopische Larynx-Fotokymografie. Bingen: R Gross Verlag.

Gross M (1993) Endoskopische Phonochirurgie in Lokalanästhesie. In: Aktuelle phoniatrisch-pädaudiologische Aspekte. Bd.1. R. Gross Verlag, 100–6.

Gross M (1998a) Diskussionsbeitrag. Berlin: Stroboskopie-Kurs.

Gross M (1998b) Endoskopische Larynx-Fotokymografie. Bingen: R. Gross Verlag.

Gurr I (1948) Untersuchungen zur Feststellung der Lage des Stimmbandes am uneröffneten Larynx. Z. Laryng. Rhinol. 27: 71.

Hacki T (1989a) Klassifizierung von Glottisdysfunktionen mit Hilfe der Elektroglottographie. Folia Phoniatr. 41: 43–8.

Hacki T (1989b) Neue Möglichkeiten der Diagnostik in der Stimmphysiologie und -pathologie mittels Sprech- und Singstimmfeldmessungen sowie der Elektroglottographie. Hannover: Habilitationsschrift.

Hacki T (1996) Electroglottographic quasi-open quotient and amplitude in crescendo phonation. J.of Voice 10: 342–7.

Hahn C. Kitzing P (1978) Indirect endoscopic photographie of the larynx. Journal of Audiovisual Media in Medicine 1: 121–30.

Harless E (1852) Stimme. In Wagners Handwörterbuch. Physiologie. 4.Bd. 673.

Harries ML, Morrison M (1996) The role of stroboscopy in the management of a patient with a unilateral fold paralysis. J.Laryng.Otol. 110(2): 141–3.

Hertz Ch, Lindström K, Sonesson B (1970) Ultrasonic recording of vibrating vocal folds: preliminary report. Acta Otolaryng. (Stockh.) 69: 223–30.

Hess MM, Gross M (1993) High-speed, light-intensified digital imaging of vocal fold vibrations in high optical resolution via indirect microlaryngoscopy. Ann Otol Rhinol Laryngol 102: 502–7.

Hess MM, Ludwigs M (2000a) Lupenlaryngoskopie und Stroboskopie mit Leuchtdioden. In M Gross (ed.), Aktuelle phoniatrisch-pädaudiologische Aspekte, Band 7. Heidelberg: Median-Verlag.

Hess MM, Ludwigs M (2000b) 'Pocket' strobe: a lightweight and battery driven laryngo-stroboscopy illumination system. Laryngo-Rhino-Otol 79(1) Suppl.: 112.

Hess MM et al. (1996) Endoskopische Darstellung von Stimmlippenschwingungen. HNO 44: 685–93.

Hess MN, Ludwigs M, Orglmeister R, Gross M (1997) Videoendoskopische Strobo-Photo-Glottographie (SPGG). In M Gross, U Eysholdt (eds), Aktuelle phoniatrisch-pädaudiologische Aspekte 1996. Bd. 4, Göttingen: Verlag Abteilung Phoniatrie, 11–12.

Hess M, Ludwigs M, Gross M (1998) Vocal fold separation pattern. In M. Gross (ed.), Aktuelle phoniatrisch-pädaudiologische Aspekte 1997/98. Band 5. Heidelberg: Median Verlag, 30–2.

Heyning, PH van de, Remacle M, Cauwenberge P, Belgian Study Group on Voice Disorders (1996) Concluding remarks. Acta oto-rhino-laryngologica belg. 50: 361–2. Appendix 1, 2, 3.

Hirano M (1974) Morphological structure of the vocal cord as vibrator and its variations. Folia phoniatrica 26(2): 89–94.

Hirano M (1989) Objective evaluation of the human voice: clinical aspects. Folia phoniatr. 41: 89–144.

Hirano M (1991) Phonosurgical anatomy of the larynx. In CN Ford, DM Bless (eds), Phonosurgery: Assessment and Surgical Management of Voice Disorders. Raven Press, New York.

Hirano M (1993) Surgical anatomy and physiology of the vocal folds. In WJ Gould, RT Sataloff, JR Spiegel (eds), Voice Surgery. St. Louis: Mosby, 135–58.

Hirano M, DM Bless (1993) Videostroboscopic Examination of the Larynx. San Diego: Singular Publishing Group.

Hirano M, Sato K (1995) Histological Color Atlas of the Human Larynx. San Diego: Singular Publishing Group.

Hirano M., Kiyikawa K, Kurita S, Sator K (1986) Posterior glottis. Morphological study in excised human larynges. Ann.Otol. Rhinol.Laryngol. 95: 576–81.

Hoefler H (1995) Larynxstroboscopie. Fortbildungskurs, Bad Gastein/Austria.

Holmer N-G, Kitzing P, Lindström K (1973) Echo glottography. Acta Otolaryng. (Stockh.) 75: 454–63.

Inagi K et al. (1997) Correlation between vocal functions and glottal measurements in patients with unilateral vocal fold paralysis. Laryngoscope 107: 782–91.

Inagi K et al. (1998) Relationship of clinical observations to objective measures in the assessment of medialization thyroplasty. Phonoscope 1(2): 85–96.

Irby KW, Hooper CR (1997) Designing a training program in laryngeal videoendostroboscopy (LVES). ASHA Convention. Boston: Poster-Session.

Iro H, Uttenweiler V (2000) Ulraschall HNO-Heilkunde. Berlin: Springer.

Isshiki N (1998) Vocal mechanics as the basis for phonosurgery. Laryngoscope 108: 1761–6.

Kahane JC (1988) Histologic structure and properties of the human voca folds. Ear Nose Throat J 67: 322–30.

Kallen LA, Polin HS (1937) Ein physiologisches Stroboskop. Mschr. Ohrenheilk. 71: 1177–81.

Kaneko T, Suziku H, Uchida K et al. (1983) The motion of the inner layers of the vocal fold during phonation-observation by ultrasonic method. In DM Bless, JH Abbs (eds), Vocal Fold Physiology: Contemporary Research and Clinical Issues. San Diego: College-Hill, 223–8.

Karduck A, Bartholomé, W (1976) Funktionelle Ergebnisse nach Radiumkontaktbestrahlung des Stimmbandkarzinoms. Laryng. Rhinol. 55: 470–7.

Karnell MP (1994) Videoendoscopy: From velopharynx to larynx. San Diego: Singular Publishing Group.

Kelsey, Ch A, Minnifie FD, Hixon TJ (1969) Applications of ultrasound in speech research. J. Speech Hear.Res. 12: 564–74.

Kitamura T, Kaneko T, Asono H (1964) Ultrasonic diagnosis of the laryngeal diseases. Jap. Med. Ultrasonics 2: 18.

Kittel G (1978) Lupen-Mikro-TV-Farbstroboskopie mit Amplitudenbestimmungs-möglichkeiten. HNO, 94–6.

Kitzing P (1985) Stroboscopy – a pertinent laryngological examination. J. of Otolaryngology 14(3): 151–7.

Kitzing P (1990) Clinical application of electroglottography. J. of Voice 4: 238–49.

Kitzing P, Sonessen B (1974) A photoglottographical study of the female vocal folds during phonation. Folia phoniat. 26: 138–49.

Kleinsasser N et al. (1994) Endoskopische, dreidimensionale Vermessung von Neubildungen und Stenosen des Larynx und der Trachea. Laryngo-Rhino-Otol. 73: 428–39.

Klingholz F, Arndt HJ (1988) Die akustische Analyse des primären Larynxtons. Sprache-Stimme-Gehör 12: 1–4.

Kokesh J et al. (1993) Correlation between stroboscopy and electromyography in laryngeal paralysis. Ann Otol Rhinol Laryngol 102: 852–7.

Kost KM, Eibling DE, Rosen CA (1996) Helpful hints in videostroboskopy. American Academy of Otolaryngology. Annual Meeting. Washington, 30 Sept. Handout.

Köster VO (1997) Stimmphysiologische Untersuchungen mittels Hochgeschwindigkeit-skinematographie. Trier: WVT Wissenschaftlicher Verlag.

Krmpotic-Nematic J, et al. (1985) Topographische Anatomie des Kopf-Halsbereiches. Munich: Urban & Schwarzenberg.

Leanderson R, Sundberg J (1988) Breathing for singing. J.of Voice 2(1): 2–12.

Leden, H v (1961) The electronic synchron-stroboscope. Ann.Otol.Rhinol. Laryng. 70: 881–93.

Leden, H v, Moore P (1961) Vibratory pattern of the vocal cords in unilateral paralysis. Arch Otolaryngol 53: 493–506.

Leden H v, Moore P, Timcke R (1960) Laryngeal vibrations: Measurements of the glottic wave. Part III. Arch. Otolaryngol. 71: 16–35.

Leder SB, Ross DA, Briskin KB, Sasaki CT (1997) A prospective, double-blind, randomized study on the use of a topical anesthetic, vasoconstrictor and placebo during transnasal flexible fiberoptic endoscopy. J. Speech Language a. Hearing Research 40: 1352–7.

Lehman JJ, Bless DM, Brandenburg JH (1988) An objective assessment of voice production after radiation therapy for stage I squamous cell carcinoma of the glottis. Otolaryngology – Head and Neck Surgery 98: 121–9.

Lehmann W et al. (1981) Larynx. Microlaryngoscopy and Histopathology. Inpharzam (Switzerland): Inpharzam Medical Publications.

Lenz R (1990) Grundlagen der Videometrie, angewandt auf eine ultra-hochauflösende CCD-Farbkamera; Technisches Messen tm 57(10): 366–80.

Ludwigs M, Hess M, Orglmeister R, Gross M (1996a) Extraktion verschiedener Parameter bei der videostroboskopischen Bildanalyse. In M Gross (ed.), Aktuelle phoniatrisch-pädaudiologische Aspekte 1995. Bd. 3. Berlin: R. Gross Verlag, 71–5.

Ludwigs M, Orglmeister R, Hess M, Gross M (1996b) Qualitätsverbesserung von videolaryngostroboskopischen Aufnahmen unter besonderer Berücksichtigung der digitalen Bildanalyse. In M Gross (ed.), Aktuelle phoniatrisch-pädaudiolgische Aspekte 1995, Band 3. Berlin: RGV-Verlag, 67–70.

Ludwigs M, Orglmeister R, Hess M (1997) Kombination von supra- und subglottischer Beleuchtung bei der Videostroboskopie. In M Gross, U Eysholdt (eds), Aktuelle phoniatrisch-pädaudiologische Aspekte 1996. Bd. 4. Göttingen: Verlag Abteilung Phoniatrie, 215–16

McKelvie P, Grey P, North C (1970) Laryngeal strobomicroscope. Lancet II: 503–4.

McLean-Muse A et al. (2000) Thyroplasty Implant for Vocal Fold Immobility: Phonatory Outcomes. Ann Otol Rhinol Laryngol 109: 393–400.

Mathieu HF, Peeters AJGE (1998) The value of videolaryngostroboscopy and videokymography in detection and imaging of early glottic carcinoma. Europ. Arch.of Oto-Rhino-Laryngol. 225, Suppl. 1: 536.

Maurer D, Hess M, Gross M (1996) High-speed imaging vocal fold vibrations and larynx movements within vocalizations of different vowels. Ann Otol Rhinol Laryngol 105: 975–81.

Mensch B (1964) Analyse par exploration ultrasonicque du mouvement des cordes vocales isolées. Comtes rendes des séances de la Société de Biologie 158: 2295–6.

Mergell P (1998) Nonlinear dynamics of Phonation-High-Speed Glottography and Biomechanical Modeling of Vocal Fold Oscillations. Aachen: Shaker Verlag.

Mergell P, Tigges M, Herzel H, Eysholdt U (1999) HGG und Modellierung von irregulären Stimmlippenschwingungen bei Larynxparesen. In M Gross (ed.), Aktuelle phoniatrisch-pädaudiologische Aspekte 1998/1999. Heidelberg: Median-Verlag, 12–17.

Miller G, Monnier Ph (1981) Lemites de la fibroscopie. Acta endoscopica Tome Nr. XI 4–5: 263–74.

Minifie FD, Kelsey CA, Hixon TJ (1968) Measurement of vocal motion using an ultrasonic Doppler velocity monitor. J.Acoust Soc Am 43: 1165–9.

Minnigerode B (1969) Das Defigurationsphänomen in der Bewegungswahrnehmung und seine Auswirkung auf das stroboskopische Kehlkopfbild. Mschr. Ohrenheilk 103: 210–17.

Miura T (1969) Mode of vocal cord vibration: a study with ultrasonoglottography. J Otolaryngol Jpn 72: 985–1002.

Murry Th, Abitbol J, Hersan R (1999) Quantitative assessment of voice quality following laser surgery for Reinke`s edema. J. of Voice 13(2): 257–64.

Musehold A (1898) Stroboskopische und photographische Studien über die Stellung der Stimmlippen im Brust- und Falsett-Register. Arch.Laryng. Rhinol. (Berl.) 7: 1–21.

Myung-Whun Sung, Kwang Hyun K, Tae-Young K et al. (1999) Videostrobokymography: a new method for the quanitative analysis of vocal fold vibration. Laryngoscope 109: 1859–63.

Naturwissenschaft und Technik (1991) Schall/Bild/Optik. Köln: Lingen Verlag.

Niimi S, Miyaji M (2000) Vocal fold vibration and voice quality. Folia Phoniatr Logop 52: 32–8.

Oertel MJ (1887) Über eine neue laryngostroboskopische, Untersuchungsmethode des Kehlkopfs'. Zentralblatt med. Wiss. 81–2(5).

Oertel MJ (1895) Das Laryngo-Stroboskop und die laryngo-stroboskopische Untersuchung. Arch. Laryng. Rhinol. 3: 1–16.

Omori K et al. (1996) Quantitative videostroboscopic measurement of glottal gap and vocal function: an analysis of thyroplasty type I. Ann.Otol. Rhinol. Laryngol. 105: 280–5.

Omori K et al. (1997) Vocal fold atrophy: quantitative glottic measurement and vocal function. Ann. Otol. Rhinol. Laryngol. 106: 544–51.

Ooi LLPJ, Chan HS, Soo KC (1995) Color doppler imaging for vocal cord palsy. Head & Neck 17(1): 20–3.

Orlikoff RF (1998) Scrambled EGG: The uses and abuses of electroglottography. Phonoscope 1(1): 37–53.

Orlikoff RF et al. (1999) Vocal function following successful chemoradiation treatment for advanced laryngeal cancer: preliminary results. Phonoscope 2(2): 66–77.

Ott S (1997) Stimm-, Sprech- und Sprachstörungen. In: Klinikleitfaden Hals-, Nasen-Ohrenheilk.2.Aufl. Fischer, Ulm/Stuttgart/Jena/Luebeck.

Pahn J, Dahl R (1995) Vorschlag einer computergestützten Datenerfassung des laryngoskopischen Befundes der Glottisfunktion. In M Gross (ed.), Aktuelle phoniatrisch-pädaudiologische Aspekte 1994. Band 2. Berlin: R. Gross Verlag, 101–4.

Pahn J, Dahl R (1996) Sprache Stimme Gehör 20: 63–5.

Panconcelli-Calzia G (1957) Über die durch Synchron-Stroboskopie neubedingten Aufgaben der Untersuchung von Vorgängen im Kehlkopf. Laryng. Rhinol. Otol. 36: 570–4.

Pascher W, Homoth R, Kruse G (1971) Verbesserte visuelle Diagnostik in der Laryngologie und Phoniatrie. HNO 19: 373–5.

Pease BC, Hoasjoe DK, Stucker FJ (1997) Videostroboscopic findings in laryngeal tuberculosis. Otolaryngology – Head and Neck Surgery 117(6): 230–4.

Poburka BJ (1999) A new stroboscopy rating form. J. of Voice 13(3): 403–13.

Poburka BJ, Bless DM (1998) A multi-media, computer-based method for stroboscopy rating training. J. of Voice 12(4): 513–26.

Postma GN, Courey MS, Ossoff RH (1998) Microvascular lesions of the true vocal fold. Ann. Otol. Rhinol. Laryngol. 107: 472–6.

Proctor DF (1980) Breathing, Speech and Song. Wien/New York: Springer.

Remacle M (1996) The contribution of videostroboscopy in daily ENT practice. Acta oto-rhino-laryngologica belg. 50: 265–81.

Remacle M, Lawson J, Keghian J, Jamart J (1999) Use of injectable autologous collagen for correcting glottis gap initial results. J. of Voice 13(2): 280–8.

Salimbeni C, Alajmo E (1985) Laryngostroboscopic observation by means of inferior glottoscopy. J. of Laryngology a. Otology 99: 801–3.

Sataloff RT (1997) Professional Voice: The Science and Art of Clinical Care, 2nd edn, San Diego/London: Singular Publishing Group.

Sataloff RT, Spiegel JR, Hawkshaw MJ (1991) Strobovideolaryngoscopy: results and clinical value. Ann. Otol. Rhinol. Laryngol. 100: 725–7.

Sato K (1998) Reticular fibers in the vocal fold mucosa. Ann. Otol. Rhinol. Laryngol. 197: 1023–8.

Schade G, Kothe C (1999) Sonoanatomie des Larynx. Ultraschall in Med. 20: 129.

Schindler O, Gonella ML, Pisani R (1990) Doppler ultrasound examination of the vibration speed of vodal folds. Folia Phoniatr 42: 265–72

Schneider B, Wendler J, Seidner W (1998) Zur Bedeutung der Stroboskopie bei der Klassifizierung funktioneller Dysphonien. HNO 46(4): 465.

Schönhärl E (1960) Die Stroboskopie in der praktischen Laryngologie. Stuttgart: Thieme.

Schröter-Morasch H (1998) Beurteilung vom Velopharynx und Larynx bei Dysarthrie. In W Ziegler, M Vogel, B Gröne, H Schröter-Morasch, Dysarthrie. Stuttgart/New York: Thieme, 53–72.

Schuerenberg B (1990) Die Beurteilung stroboskopischer Kriterien. Folia phoniatr. 42: 41–8.

Schultz-Coulon H-J (1980) Die Diagnostik der gestörten Stimmfunktion. Arch. Otorhinolaryngol. 227: 1–169.

Schultz-Coulon H-J (1982) Physiologie und Untersuchungsmethoden des Kehlkopfes. In v Berendes et al. (eds), Hals-Nasen-Ohren-Heilkunde in Praxis und Klinik. 2. Aufl. Band 4, Teil 1: Kehlkopf 1. Stuttgart/New York: Thieme.

Schutte HK, Svec JG (1994) Video-Kymography – a modern imaging system for analyzing regular and irregular vocal fold vibrations. Proc. XXth Congr. Collegium Medicom Theatri, Santa Fe NM.

Schutte HK, Svec JG, Sram F (1998) First results of clinical application of videokymography. Laryngoscope 108: 1206–10.

Scope View (1998) Dr. Speech. Software. Seattle: Tiger Electronics.

Seeman M (1921) Laryngostroboskopische Untersuchungen bei einseitiger Rekurrensparese. Mschr. Ohrenheilk. 55: 1621–34.

Seidner W, Wendler J (1997) Die Sängerstimme, 3. Aufl. Berlin: Henschel Verlag.

Seidner W, Wendler J (2000) Indirekte Mikrophonochirurgie. HNO-Informationen 24(2): 127.

Seidner W, Wendler J, Halbedel G (1972) Mikrostroboskopie. Folia phoniat. 24: 81–5.

Sercarz JA et al. (1991) A new technique for qualitative measurement of laryngeal videostroboscopic images. Arch. Otolaryngol. Head Neck Surg. 117: 871–5.

Sercarz JA et al. (1992) Videostroboscopy of human vocal fold paralysis. Ann.Otol. Rhinol.Laryngol. 101: 567–77.

Sessions RB et al. (1992) Videolaryngostroboscopy for evaluation of laryngeal disorders. In A Blitzer et al. (eds), Neurologic Disorders of the Larynx. Stuttgart: Thieme.

Sonessen B (1960) On the anatomy and vibrator pattern of the human vocal folds. Acta oto-laryng. (Stockh.), Suppl. 156: 7–80.

Sonessen B (1962) Photo-electric demonstration of the vibratory movements of the human vocal folds. Proc. XII. Intern. Speech Voice Ther. Conf., 57–61.

Sopko J (1980) Funktionelle Ergebnisse nach Bestrahlung des Larynxkarzinoms. In Aktuelle Probleme der Otorhinolaryngologie 3. Bd. 3. Bern/Stuttgart/Wien: H. Huber, 80–6.

Sovák M (1945a) Kmitáni hlasivek ve svetle laryngostroboskopie [Vocal fold vibration in the light of laryngostroboscopy] (In Czech). Prague: Ceská akademie ved a umeni.

Sovák M (1945b) Stroboskopický výzkum hlasové pathologie: Studie o poruchách fonacniho mechanismu. [Stroboscopic research of voice pathology: A study on the disorders of the phonation mechanism] (In Czech). Prague: Ceská akademie ved a umeni.

Spiegel JR, Sataloff RT, Hawkshaw M, Rosen DC (1996) Vocal fold hemorrhage. Ear Nose and Throat J. 75(12): 784–9.

Spiesberger W, Tasto M (1981) Processing of medical image sequences. In TS Huang (ed.), Image Sequence Analysis, Springer Series in Information Science, Berlin: Springer.

Šram F, Švec JG (2000) Results of videokymographic examinations by functional voice disorders. In M Gross (ed.), Aktuelle phoniatrisch-pädaudiologische Aspekte 1998/1999, Band 6. Heidelberg: Median-Verlag.

Šram F, Švec JG, Schutte HK (1999) Possibilities for use of videokymography in laryngologic and phoniatric practice. In PH Dejonckere, HFM Peters (eds), Proceedings 24th IALP Congress. Amsterdam, 1998. Vol. I. Nijmegen University Press, pp. 256–9.

Štelzig Y̌, Hochaus W, Gall V, Henneberg A (1999) Kehlkopfbefunde bei Patienten mit Morbus Parkinson. Laryngo-Rhino-Otol. 78: 544–55.

Stemple JC, Gerdemann BK, Kelchner LN (1998) Instrumental measurement of voice. In JC Stemple et al. (eds), Clinical Voice Pathology. San Diego: Singular Publishing Group.

Story BH, Titze JR (1995) Voice simulation with a body-cover model of the vocal folds. J. Acoust. Soc. Am. 97(2): 1249–60.

Stuckrad H v, Lakatos L (1974) Eine neue endoskopische Methode zur Diagnostik und Fotodokumentation von Larynx und Hypopharynx. Arch. Ohr -, Nas- u. Kehlk.-Heilk. 207: 549–50.

Stuckrad H v, Lakatos L (1975) Über ein neues Lupenlaryngoskop (Epipharyngoskop). Laryng. Rhinol. 54: 336–40.

Suzuki H, Kaneko T, Numata T et al. (1986) Newly developed ultrasound laryngographic equipment and 1st clinical application. In Proceedings of the XXth Congress Intern. Association Logopedics and Phoniatrics, Tokyo, 366–7.

Švec JG, Schutte HK (1996) Videokymography: high-speed line scanning of vocal fold vibration. J. of Voice 10(2): 201–5.

Švec JG, Sram F, Schutte HK (1999) Videokymography: a new high-speed method for the examination of vocal-fold vibrations (Czech). Otorinolaryngol. (Prague), 48(3): 155–62.

Tigges M, Wittenberg T, Rosanowski F, Eysholdt U (1996) Bildsegmentierung zur quantitativen Auswertung von laryngoskopischen Videoaufnahmen. In M Gross (ed.), Aktuelle phoniatrisch-pädaudiologische Aspekte 1995 5, Band 3. Berlin: R. Gross Verlag, 65–6.

Tigges M et al. (1998) Functional voice disorders – a non-linear system? Possible uses of quantitative laryngoscopy. Eur. Arch.Oto-Rhino-Laryng. 225(1): 33–4.

Timcke R (1956) Die Synchron-Stroboskopie von menschlichen Stimmlippen bzw. ähnlichen Schallquellen und Messung der öffnungszeit. Z. Laryng. Rhinol. 35: 331–5.

Timcke R, Leden H v, Moore P (1958) Laryngeal vibrations: measurements of the glottic wave. Part I. The normal vibratory cycle. Arch. Otolaryngol. 68: 1–19.

Timcke R, Leden H v, Moore P (1959) Laryngeal vibrations: measurements of the glottic wave. Part II. Physiologic variations. Arch. Oto-laryngol. 69: 438–44.

Titze IR (1994) Principles of Voice Production. Englewood Cliffs: Prentice-Hall.

Titze IR (1998) The voice chain: from protein to tissue to sound. Special Session. ASHA Annual Convention, San Antonio, Nov. 1998.

Tonndorf W (1929) Zur Physiologie des menschlichen Stimmorgans. Z. Hals-, Nasen- u. Ohrenheilkunde 22: 412–23.

Töpler (1866) Poggendorfs Ann. Physik u. Chemie 128: 108.

Tsunoda K et al. (1997) Stroboscopic observation of the larynx after radiation in patients with T 1 glottic carcinoma. Acta Otolaryngol. (Stockh.) Suppl. 527: 165–6.

Uttenweiler V (2000) Funktionelle Ultraschalldiagnostik. In H Iro, V Uttenweiler, J Zenk, Kopf-Hals-Sonographie. Berlin: Springer, 97–110.

Vallancien B (1957) Stroboskopic et télévision. J. franc. d'Oto-Rhino-Laryngologie 6(3): 418–20.

Wallesch B, Sieron J, Johannsen HS (1991) Über die Wertigkeit der indirekten Mikrolaryngoskopie in der Nachsorge von Patienten mit primär radiierten Stimmlippenkarzinomen. Laryngo-Rhinol-Otol. 70: 559–61.

Ward PH, Berci G, Calcaterra TC (1974) Advances in endoscopic examination of the respiratory system. Ann. Otol. Rhinol. 83: 754–60.

Watanabe H et al. (1986) A new computer-analyzing system for clinical use with a strobo-videoscope. Arch. Otolaryng. Head Neck Surg. 112: 978–81.

Weise W, Quattrocchi P (1983) Informations- und Codierungstheorie: Mathematische Grundlagen der Datenkompression und -Sicherung in diskreten Kommunikationssystemen. Berlin: Springer Verlag.

Weiss D (1932) Die Laryngostroboskopie. Zschr. Laryng.Rhinol.Otol. 22: 391–418.

Wendler J (1976) Practical hints for the application of laryngostroboscopy. VEB Transformation- und Röntgenwerke. Dresden.

Wendler J (1983) Indirect microsurgery of the vocal folds under functional control. Proc. XIX congr. IALP, Vol. III, 928–30.

Wendler J (1997) Laryngeal stroboscopy. Instruction course. Sydney 1997. XVI World Congress of Otorhinolaryngology Head and Neck Surgery. 2–7 March. Abstract book, p. 18.

Wendler J, Köppen K (1988) Schwingungsmessungen der Stimmlippen: Zur klinischen Relevanz der Stroboskopie. Folia Phoniatr. 40: 297–302.

Wendler J, Otto C, Nawka T (1983) Stroboglottometrie – ein neues Verfahren zur Schwingungsanalyse der Stimmlippen. Leipzig: HNO-Praxis, 8, 263–8.

Wendler J, Seidner W, Halbedel G, Schaaf G (1973) Tele-Mikrostroboskopie. Folia phoniat. 25: 281–7.

Wendler J, Seidner W, Kittel G, Eysholdt U (1996) Lehrbuch der Phoniatrie und Pädaudiologie, 3. Aufl., Stuttgart/New York: Thieme.

Wittenberg T (1998) Wissensbasierte Bewegungsanalyse von Stimmlippen schwingungen anhand digitaler Hochgeschwindigkeitsaufnahmen. Aachen: Shaker Verlag.

Wittenberg T, Mergell P, Tigges M, Eysholdt U (1998) Extraktion und Auswertung digitaler High-Speed-Kymogramme von Stimmlippenschwingungen. In M Gross (ed.), Aktuelle phoniatrisch-pädaudiologische Aspekte 1997/98. Band 5. Heidelberg: Median Verlag, 25–9.

Woo P (1996) Quantification of videostrobolaryngoscopic findings-measurements of the normal glottal cycle. Laryngoscope. Suppl. 79: 1–20.

Woo P (1997) Clinical applications of videostroboscopy in voice disorders. Current Opinion in Otolaryngology & Head and Neck Surgery 5: 133–9.

Woo P, Colton R, Casper J, Brewer D (1991) Diagnostic value of stroboscopic examination in hoarse patients. J. of Voice 5: 231–8.

Woodson GE (1993) Configuration of the glottis in laryngeal paralysis. I: Clinical study. Laryngoscope 103: 1227–34; II: Animal experiments Laryngoscope 103: 1235–41

Yanagisawa E (1982a) Effektive photographie in otolaryngology-head and neck surgery: Tympanic membrane photographie. Otolaryngol. Head, Neck Surg. 90: 399–407.

Yanagisawa E (1982b) Office telescopic photographie of the larynx. Ann. Otol. Rhinol. Laryngol. 91: 354–8.

Yoshida Y (1979) A video-tape recording system for laryngostroboscopy. J. Jap. Bronchoesoph. Soc. 30: 6–12.

Zagzebski JA, Bless DM, Ewanowski SJ (1983) Pulse echo imaging of the larynx using rapid ultrasonic scanners. In DM Bless, JH Abbs (eds), Vocal Fold Physiology: Contemporary Research and Clinical Issues. San Diego: College-Hill: 210–22.

Zappia F, Campani R (2000) The larynx: an anatomical and functional echographic study. Radiol Med (Torino) 99(3): 138–44.

Zeitels SM, Hillman RE, Bunting GW, Vaughn T (1997) Reinke's edema: phonatory mechanisms and management strategies. Ann. Otol. Rhinol. Laryngol. 106: 533–43.

Zhao R, Hirano M, Tanaka S, Sato K (1991) Vocal fold epithelial hyperplasia. Vibratory behavior vs extent of lesion. Arch. Otolaryngol. Head Neck Surgery 117: 1015–18.

Current
Equipment

Demuth Elektronik

Type designation . . . . Laryngostroboskop automatic
Address . . . . Neuengammer Hausdeich 491c
. . . . 21037 Hamburg Germany
Telephone 0049 40 7233491
Fax 0049 40 7233142
E-Mail . . . . demuthelektronik@t-online.de
Internet . . . . www. demuthelektronik.de

Technical Specifications of the Basic unit
Functional principle of the stroboscopic unit . . . . 2 lamps - flash - light and permanent light
flash bulb . . . . xenonox short-arc
brightness . . . . 6000 lm
economic life time . . . . about 5 years when using every day
halogenlamp . . . . 6000 lm 150w
brightness . . . . see above
economic life time . . . . 300 hours
filter for colour temperature . . . . yes
Step down ration of the flash lamps 600–1200Hz 1:2, 75–600Hz 1:1

Technical Specifications of the video camera
one chip- or three chip camera . . . . one chip CCD 752H, 582V
automatic white balance . . . . yes
autoclave safe . . . . in part
weight . . . . 48 g
external dimensions . . . . diameter 18 mm, length 32 mm
camera thread (C-Mount) . . . . by request
sensitivity (Lux) . . . . 2 Lux with f= 5,6
endoscope adapter . . . . 36 mm
closure mechanism . . . . clip
focus . . . . adjustable
mark for an orthograde adjustment of the endoscope . . yes
foot switch for still and moved picture . . . . yes 0°–400°
settling time of the microphone control . . . . first half wave
insertion of additional data . . . . sound level dB(A) frequency Hz

Microphone
ball characteristic . . . . yes
alignment characteristic . . . . by request
body sound microphone with bracket . . . . by request
airborne sound microphone . . . . yes
determination of fundamental frequency
    via electroglottography . . . . optional
fixation of the microphone . . . . on the endoscope
recommended endoscopes . . . . regide and flexible endoscops
picture documentation (video recorder/digital) . . . . digital 80 GBit
type of the video recorder . . . . Sony S-VHS
type of the computer system . . . . rp Szene
possibility of an additional labelling of the
    recorded pictures . . . . via rp Szene
type of monitor . . . . sony
trolley . . . . yes
other accessories . . . . camera holder, endoscop holder

Advantages of the complete system in the opinion of the manufacturer

The Laryngostroboscope Demuth automatic is a fully automatic appliance. There are no buttons to adjust the filters and the sensitiveness of the microphone. The tone phonated by the patient is recorded by a small airborne sound microphone Ø 10 mm which is fixed to the endoscope or to the patients collar. For the recording on the video-stroboscopic this tone will be given out by a socket of the appliance, as well as the basic frequency (fo) and the sound pressure in dB (A). This is only valid for appliances with installed fade-in of the measured values. The formation of the basic frequency happens within the instrument without delay at 440 Hz and needs less than 20 ms at 120 Hz. The flash needs about 5 ms. These values produce an excellent and sharply defined picture. It is also possible to synchronise using a microphone fixed to the body. In this case the larynx could be gently displaced by the pressure of the contact surface.

It is economical to use separate Xenon-lamps for the flash-light and the permanent light. The differences in the colour-temperature which may occur are compensated by filters. You work with a pedal > stop – still 0-400° – slow motion 0.75 Hz <. You can double the frequency of the slow motion by pressing a button at the appliance. The speed of the slow motion may also adjust on other values between 0 and 2 Hz.

There is a second light exit to connect for example a head lamp or in case of lamp defect, to finish the examination. An installed ON/OFF-Airflow helps prevent the optic becoming clouded.

A camera-head of high luminous intensity with digital zoom 1:3 makes a full image size possible without changing the lens using thin flexible endosopes.

Engineering data
- Reduction   70 bis 600 Hz 1: 1, 600 bis 1200 Hz 1:2
- Slow motion frequency 0 to 2 Hz, fix 0,75 and 1,5 Hz
- Still   phase deplacement 0-400°
- Microphone control   0 to max. 20 ms.
- Frequency indication self-shining display, height of the digits 13 mm
- Data issue   tone, basic frequency (fo)
- Lamps   Xenophot and Xenon small curvature lamp 150W
- 2 lightoutput   Xenophot 150 W, digitally adjustable
- Airflow   1,5 Litres / min
- AC mains input   230 V ~
- Power input   max. 340 W
- Size   B 385 mm, H 128 mm, D 295 mm
- Weight   13 Kg
- Security norm   Œ
- Classification   after MPG I

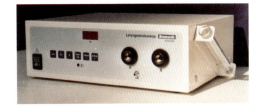

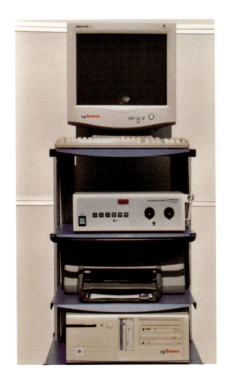

PULSAR® Stroboscope

Company Adress	KARL STORZ GmbH & Co. KG
. . . .	Mittelstr. 8
. . . .	78532 Tuttlingen / Germany
Phone:	+49 7461 708 0
Fax:	+49 7461 708 105
E-mail:	info@karlstorz.de
Internet:	www.karlstorz.de

Specifications:

Power supply voltage:	100 – 125 / 220 – 240 VAC; 50/60 Hz
Power consumption:	340 VA
Strobe light output:	2.5 Ws (impulse energy)
Triggerable frequency range:	80 – 1400 Hz
Strobe frequency (variable):	min. 50 – max. 200 Hz
Slow motion frequency:	0.5 – 2,5 Hz
Phase difference:	0 – 400°
Additional light source, continous:	Halogen 150 W/15 V
Insufflation pump (flow performance):	2 l/min.
Dimensions:	450 x 155 x 320 mm (w x h x d)
Weight:	24 kg
Microphone:	Airborne sound microphone

Conformity to IEC 601-1 Standards

Type of protection against electrical shock: . . .	Protection Class 1
Degree of protectionagainst electrical shock: . .	Type BF device
Medical Device Directive (MDD):	93/42/EEC

Recommended Telescopes . . . . **KARL STORZ** *Hopkins* **Telescopes** for Laryngo- / Pharyngoscopy

. . . .	8705 CKA 70°, diameter 4 mm
. . . .	8706 CA 70°, diameter 7.2 x 9.3 mm
. . . .	8700 CKA 70°, diameter 5.8 mm
. . . .	8700 DKA 90°, diameter 5.8 mm
. . . .	8707 DA 90°, diameter 10 mm

Recommended Fiberscope . . . . **KARL STORZ Laryngo-Fiberscope**

. . . .	11101 RP1 diameter 3.7 mm, length 30 cm

Technical Specification of the KARL STORZ TELECAM® Camera System

Image sensor:	½" CCD chip
Pixel:	752 (H) x 582 (V) pixel (PAL) 768 (H) x 494 (V) pixel (NTSC)
Resolution:	> 450 lines (horizontal)
Signal-/noise ratio:	> 50 dB (PAL) > 52 dB (NTSC)
AGC:	+ 18 dB
Min. sensitivity:	3 Lux (f=1.4)
Lens:	Separate C-mount lens, f = 12 mm, f = 25 mm, f = 30 mm
. . . .	or f = 38 mm
Instrument coupling:	Coupling device for all rigid and flexible endoscopes with
. . . .	standard eyepiece
Video output:	Composite signal to BNC socket, Y/C signal to S-VHS socket
. . . .	(2 x)
Control output:	3.5 mm stereo jack plug (ACC 1, ACC 2)
Camera head:	Dimensions: diameter 28 – 43 mm, length 51 mm
Weight:	80 g
Camera cable:	Length: 300 cm
Camera Control Unit (CCU): Dimensions:	305 x 89 x 335 mm (w x h x d)
Weight:	2.95 kg
Certified to:	IEC 601-1, 601-2-18, CSA 22.2 no. 601, UL 2601
. . . .	and CE in accordance with MDD, Protection Class 1/BF

With only one bulb, the KARL STORZ PULSAR stroboscope produces high performance XENON light for stroboscoping (pulsating light), as well as for normal observation (continuous light).
A special trigger technique prevents effects, such as drop outs, hovering and modulations in brightness.

The advantages of this system are:

- No mechanical / optical elements for the changeover between strobe light and continuous light, therefore, no darkness phase
- No difference in the color temperature between strobe light and continuous light
- No difference in the brightness between strobe light and continuous light
- Modular construction simplifies the addition of optional functions
- Compact design
- Simple user interface
- Integrated insufflation pump

The range of functions for the device can be expanded with the following options:

- Loudspeaker for the output of the pilot tone (electrical tuning fork)
- Keyboard for text input or with card reader device (only available in Germany)
- Head light holder with switch function (to activate additional light source)
- Control function for video recorder (only with video module)

When combined with an optional video module additional functions are available:

- Automatic brightness control
- Text and data can be displayed in the video image
- Control of a video recorder

Further advantages are available when combined with an optional halogen second light source:

- Economical halogen light for standard applications
- Separate light output for connection to a second light-transmitting instrument
- No additional space requirement
- No additional operation field

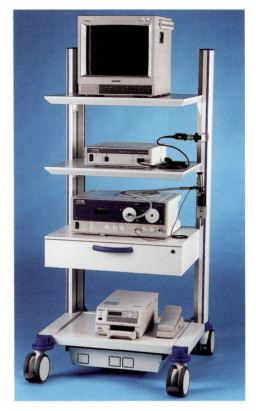

Due to the modular system design, all of the options are simple to implement. This advantage is particularly valuable for exchanging the strobe light or when re-equipping the halogen second light source. As a result, it is possible to change the module/light:

- directly at the location where the system is being used without having to remove the device from the equipment cart
- practical to implement, as only a few parts need to be disassembled
- no adjustment of the light is required
- no special safety measures are required (apart from disconnecting from the mains power supply)

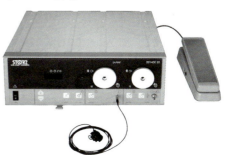

ATMOS MedizinTechnik

Type designation . . . . Endo-Stroboscope L
Company . . . . ATMOS MedizinTechnik GmbH & Co. KG,
Address . . . . Ludwig-Kegel-Str. 16,
                                              79853 Lenzkirch/Germany
Telephone . . . . +49 7653 689-0
Fax . . . . +49 7653 689-392 (national)
                                              +49 7653 689-391 (international)
E-Mail . . . . atmos@atmosmed.de
Internet . . . . www. atmosmed.de

Technical Specifications
Functional principle of the stroboscopic unit . . . . light flashes
flash bulb . . . . xenon
brightness . . . . 0,7 J/flash (this is 30 times more than the 180 W
                                              xenon bulb)
economic life time . . . . > 1000 h flashlight
pilot light . . . . with flash bulb
brightness . . . . see above
economic life time . . . . see above
filter for colour temperature . . . . not necessary in this system
gear reduction of the flash lamp in the
relation 1:1 in the aera from/to . . . . 70 up to 500 Hz
gear reduction of the flash lamp in the
relation 1:2 in the area from/to . . . . 500 up to 1000 Hz

Technical Specifications of the video camera
one chip- or three chip camera . . . . one chip camera (CCD 1/2") 440.000 pixel
automatic white balance . . . . alternatively automatic/manual, three different
                                              profiles can be stored
autoclave safe . . . . no
weight . . . . approx. 20 g (head without cable)
external dimensions . . . . diameter 17 mm, length 42 mm
camera thread (C-Mount) . . . . 15,5 x 0,5 mm incl. C-mount-adapter
sensitivity (Lux) . . . . 5 Lux with f= 1,4
endoscope adapter . . . . 4 versions available
                                              (F = 22 mm and f = 30 mm focusable)
closure mechanism . . . . one-hand operation (different versions)
focus . . . . see above
mark for an orthograde adjustment of
the endoscope . . . . yes
foot switch for production of a freezed image
or a moved picture . . . . yes
adjustment of synthesiser possible . . . . no
settling time of the microphone control . . . . < 200 ms
fade in of additional data . . . . basic frequency, sound pressure level, musical tone
                                              pitch, class of loudness (optionally)

Microphone
ball characteristic . . . . yes
alignment characteristic . . . . no
body sound microphone with bracket . . . . yes
airborne sound microphone . . . . yes
determination of fundamental frequency
via electroglottography . . . . no
fixation of the microphone . . . . fixed at the endoscope
recommended endoscopes . . . . all types possible
picture documentation (video recorder/digital) . . . . digital, alternatively analogue (video recorder)
type of the video recorder . . . . Sony S-VHS
type of the computer system . . . . ATMOS MediaStroboscope
possibility of an additional labelling of the
recorded pictures . . . . yes
type of monitor . . . . several types available
trolley . . . . several trolleys available
additional accessories . . . . voice and speech analysis software incl. voice area
options . . . . video outlet for computer picture

Advantages of the complete system in the opinion of the manufacturer

The ATMOS Endo-Stroboscope L is a well-established, user-friendly compact unit for the larynx diagnostic. It is characterised especially by the exact synchronization of the flash light and the quick display of frequency as well as its high reliability. The easy operation of the unit is done by a foot controller, herewith the slow-motion-speed from 0,5 – 2 Hz and the phase range of the stand-still picture from 0° up to 400° is adjustable. Thanks to a high light performance the ATMOS Endo-Stroboscope L is suitable especially for the video stroboscopy respectively the MediaStroboscope. An anti-fogging airflow which can be activated if required completes the user-friendly configuration.

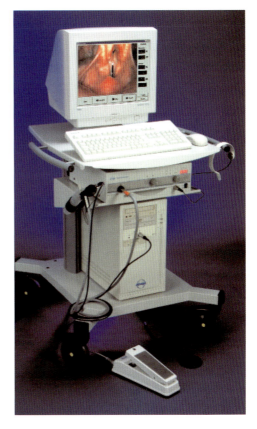

With the MediaStroboscope ATMOS offers a system especially developed for phoniatry for the digital video documentation. The video sequences of the stroboscopic examination are digitised in real time and are stored in combination with the patient data. The camera module with high resolving CCD pen-sized camera is integrated in the media workstation and corresponds to degree of protection BF of the endoscopy rule IEC 601-2-18. A data base administers patient data, examination dates and findings and plays the requested sequence very quickly and in a high quality. The spooling and rewinding of a video cassette is herewith obsolete. The voice basic frequency, sound pressure level, musical tone pitch and the class of loudness are shown as actual value and as average value and are stored together with the video data on the hard disk of the medical computer. Point and click and the requested video clip is exported into an optionally available speech and voice analysis software. The complete system is in line with the European Directive 93/42/EEC for medical products and is labelled with the corresponding CE label.

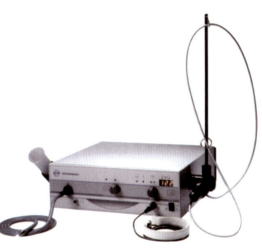

Richard Wolf GmbH

Type designation .... STROBE VIEW 5570
Company .... Richard Wolf GmbH
Address .... Pforzheimer Straße 32
                                      D-75438 Knittlingen
Telephone .... +49 7043 35-0
Fax .... +49 7043 35-300
E-Mail .... info@richard-wolf.com
Internet .... www.richard-wolf.com

Technical Specifications
Controller:
Functional principle of the stroboscopic unit .. shutter technique
Flash bulb .... no
Filter for colour temperature .... not necessary in this system
Measuring range of voice frequency .... 50 – 888 Hz
Beat time (slow motion) .... 0.5 – 2.0 sec.
Phase displacement .... 0 – 720° (with footswitch)
Noise level .... max. 50 dB(A)
Signal-to-noise-ratio .... > 50 dB
Colour control .... button for automatic white balance
Brightness control .... automatic shutter control

Camera head:
Type of camera .... one chip camera with $\frac{1}{2}$" CCD
Autoclave safe .... no
Weight .... approx. 235 g (head with cable)
External dimensions .... diameter 29 mm, length 60 mm
Camera threat .... C-mount, incl. C-mount adapter

Microphone:
Ball characteristic .... yes
Alignment characteristic .... no
Body sound microphone .... yes
Airborne sound microphone .... yes
Fixation of the microphone .... fixed at the endoscope
   Determination of the basic frequency
via electroglottography .... no

Accessories
Recommended light-source .... min. 180 W xenon
Recommended endoscopes .... all types possible
Picture documentation .... digital, alternatively analogue video recorder
.... Digital medical Cd-recorder (Motion L-Cap)
.... for capturing video sequences
Type of monitor .... several types available
Trolley .... several trolleys available

The Richard Wolf STROBE VIEW 5570 is a video stroboscope camera of the latest generation. This system introduces a new quality in the diagnosis of voice disorders. Both in terms of the value of the diagnosis and its user friendliness, the system sets new standards.

The shutter technology achieves the highest image quality and is particularly user friendly.

The STROBE VIEW 5570 can be used universally just like a "normal" endocamera. This technical concept has several extremely beneficial aspects for the customer.

The STROBE VIEW 5570 can be used in 3 modes. The changeover between modes is simple and convenient at the touch of a footswitch:

• Stroboscope mode with "slow motion"
• Stroboscope mode with "still image"
• "Normal" camera mode

The mode and phonation frequency are conveniently superimposed on the video image by the on screen display.

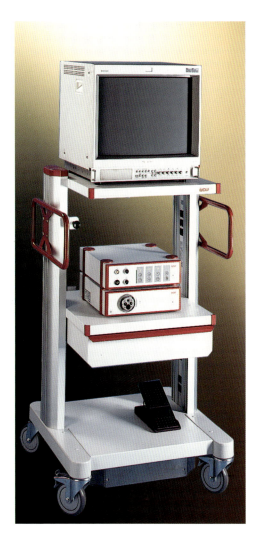

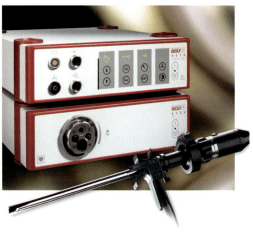

XION GmbH

Type . . . . EndoSTROB DX
Name of the company . . . . XION GmbH
Address . . . . Pankstrasse 8 – 10, 13127 Berlin, Germany
Phone . . . . +49 – 30 – 47 49 87 0
Fax . . . . +49 – 30 – 47 49 87 11
e-mail . . . . info@xion-medical.com
homepage . . . . www.xion-medical.com

Technical specification of the light source
Function principal of the stroboscopic unit . . . shutter stroboscope
Lamp . . . . continuous light, 50 watt micro-discharge lamp
Economic life time . . . . approx. 800 h
Colour temperature . . . . 6,000 K

Technical specification of the video camera
Sensor . . . . 1/3" CCD chip
Pixel . . . . 752 (H) x 582 (V) pixel (PAL)
. . . . 768 (H) x 494 (V) pixel (NTSC)
Resolution . . . . 470 lines, horizontal
420 lines, vertical
Video outputs . . . . S-Video, Video, VGA, IEEE 1394 (MPEG-2, DV)
Video inputs . . . . VGA
Illumination min. . . . . 3 lux at F 1.4
camera head . . . . 18-pin camera head with integrated microphone and
. . . . incorporated video adapter with clip coupling
Dimension . . . . 90 mm x 312 mm x 312 mm
Weight . . . . 7.1 Kg
Applied standards . . . . IEC 601 – ½, CE accoring to MDD DIN EN ISO
. . . . 13485:2001 MDD, directive 93/42 EEC

Technical specification of the stroboscope
Frequency range . . . . 80 Hz – 1,000 Hz
Slow motion . . . . 0.5 Hz – 2 Hz
Phase resolution . . . . 0° - 360°
Lock-on time . . . . < 300 ms
Operatinog modes . . . . slow motion, stationary phase

Recommended Endoscopes
Laryngoscopes . . . . Laryngoscope, Ø 7mm, 70°, Art. 130 307 427
. . . . Zoom-Laryngoscope, Ø 10mm, 70°, Art. 130 310 627
. . . . Zoom-Laryngoscope, Ø 10mm, 90°, Art. 130 310 629
Video Laryngoscope . . . . Video Laryngoscope, Ø 10mm, 70°, Art. 327 310 070
. . . . Video Laryngoscpe, Ø 10mm, 90°, Art. 327 310 090
Nasopharyngoscope . . . . Nasopharyngoscope EF-NS, Ø 3.4mm, Art. 130 400 134

EndoSTROB D –

The New Generation

The new, digital-generation system EndoSTROB D makes it possible to process and archive captured video data using all digital storage media; it is thus capable of meeting all future challenges.

- Light, compact camera head
- Integral microphone
- Sharp images with clear depiction of vocal cord margins
- Excellent colour rendering with no deviations during stroboscopy

- Light weight and compact construction, providing space-saving solutions for instrument trolleys or wall mounting
- Automatic regulation of light intensity
- Noiseless electronic stroboscope effect
- Automatic rapid detection of basal frequency
- Frequency and loudness displayed on monitor
- Interface for external regulation allows optimal integration into investigation and treatment units
- FireWire interface for digital onward transmission of video/audio data
- Simple, high-quality documentation of findings using DiVAS

Stroboscopy without a stroboscope
Unlike traditional flashlight stroboscopes, the EndoSTROB D uses continuous cold-light illumination. The stroboscopic effect is achieved by digital regulation of the camera.

Rapid recognition of frequency
The microphone incorporated in the camera head provides for reproducible recording and minimises extraneous sounds. A digital algorithm recognises the basal frequency and synchronises the camera electronics, even in the presence of high jitter or shimmer. The speed and phase of the vocal cord movements in the video picture are simple to regulate using the footpedal. This allows all the stroboscopic characteristics to be conveniently assessed: glottis closure, amplitude of oscillation, symmetry, periodicity, regularity, marginal shift of the mucosal wave, phonatory arrest, direction of vertical oscillation, and supraglottic associated vibrations.

Totally digital
Transmission direct to your computer, via a FireWire interface. This allows rapid, uncomplicated, high-quality preparation, evaluation and documentation of your findings – preferably using DiVAS, the powerful software from XION. This opens up new possibilities including computerassisted voice analysis, or subsequent comparisons with other analyses, evaluation and archiving of your findings.

Beneficial for patients
Above all, modern technology provides benefits to your patients. The camera electronics automatically regulate the intensity of the light source, thus reducing tissue heat exposure to a minimum. Unpleasant and upsetting flash-light storms are a thing of the past. The light weight and compact construction of the camera head make it safe and convenient to handle.

DiVAS

Software for Images and Video

Digital management, evaluation and archiving
Powerful software is an essential prerequisite for the rapid and efficient exploitation of your findings for diagnosis and treatment. DiVAS provides you with all the professional tools you need, and its user-friendly and intuitive user interface inspires confidence. In many different languages.

Advantages of DiVAS:
- Full image mode
- Integrated cutting options
- Free choice of single frames to identify a stored video
- Storage of computer data using MPEG-2 compression
- A variety of options for exporting image data for use in documentation
- Navigation and selection in videos using time ruler
- Input as digital video or MPEG-2 via FireWire
- Support for PAL and NTSC video systems
- Compatible with Windows XP

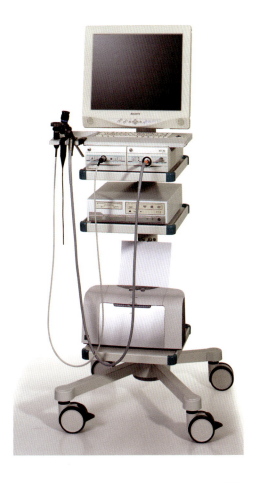

Index